PROGRESS IN CLINICAL AND BIOLOGICAL RESEARCH

RECENT TITLES

Please contact the publisher for information about previous titles in this series.

CARCINOMA OF THE LARGE BOWEL AND ITS PRECURSORS

CARCINOMA OF THE LARGE BOWEL AND ITS PRECURSORS

Proceedings of a Conference
held in Detroit, September 27–28, 1984

Editors

John R.F. Ingall
Department of Surgery
Wayne State University
Detroit, Michigan

Anthony J. Mastromarino
National Large Bowel Cancer Project
M.D. Anderson Hospital and Tumor Institute
Houston, Texas

ALAN R. LISS, INC. • NEW YORK

Address all Inquiries to the Publisher
Alan R. Liss, Inc., 41 East 11th Street, New York, NY 10003

Copyright © 1985 Alan R. Liss, Inc.

Printed in the United States of America.

Library of Congress Cataloging in Publication Data

Conference on Carcinoma of the Large Bowel and Its
    Precursors (1984 : Detroit, Mich.)
    Carcinoma of the large bowel and its precursors.

    Includes bibliographies and index.
    1. Intestine, Large—Cancer—Congresses.
2. Intestine, Large—Cancer—Etiology—Congresses.
3. Precancerous conditions—Congresses. I. Ingall,
John R.F. II. Mastromarino, Anthony J. III. Title.
[DNLM: 1. Intestinal Neoplasms—congresses. 2. Intestine,
Large—congresses. 3. Precancerous Conditions—congresses.
W1 PR668E v. 186 / WI 435 C748c 1984]
RC280.I5C66 1984   616.99′436   85-9734
ISBN 0-8451-5036-7

Contents

Contributors

David A. Ahlquist, Division of Gastro-enterology, Mayo Clinic, Rochester, MN **[45]**

Jean-Claude Bayle, Department of Surgery, Memorial Sloan-Kettering Cancer Center, New York City, NY **[1]**

John H. Bowers, Division of Gastroenterology, Departments of Surgery and Medicine, University of Utah School of Medicine, Salt Lake City, UT **[151]**

Randall W. Burt, Departments of Surgery and Medicine, University of Utah School of Medicine, Salt Lake City, UT **[151]**

William W.L. Chang, Department of Pathology, West Virginia University School of Medicine and University Hospital, Morgantown, WV **[217]**

Neal K. Clapp, Marmoset Research Program, Medical and Health Sciences Division, Oak Ridge Associated Universities, Oak Ridge, TN **[247]**

Jerome J. DeCosse, Department of Surgery, Memorial Sloan-Kettering Cancer Center, New York, NY **[1]**

Eleanor E. Deschner, Laboratory of Digestive Tract Carcinogenesis, Memorial Sloan-Kettering Cancer Center, New York, NY **[187]**

John A. Dixon, Division of Gastroenterology, Departments of Surgery and Medicine, University of Utah School of Medicine, Salt Lake City, UT **[151]**

Gerald D. Dodd, Department of Diagnostic Imaging, M.D. Anderson Hospital, Houston, TX **[133]**

Cecilia M. Fenoglio, Laboratory Services, Veterans Administration Medical Center; Department of Pathology, University of New Mexico School of Medicine, Albuquerque, NM **[23]**

Martin Fleisher, Department of Clinical Chemistry, Memorial Sloan-Kettering Cancer Center, New York, NY **[57]**

Eileen A. Friedman, Department of Gastrointestinal Cancer Research, Memorial Sloan-Kettering Cancer Center, New York, NY **[175]**

William G. Friend, Department of Surgery, University of Washington, Seattle, WA **[65]**

Barbara L. Gangaware, Marmoset Research Program, Medical and Health Sciences Division, Oak Ridge Associated Universities, Oak Ridge, TN **[247]**

Marsha A. Henke, Marmoset Research Program, Medical and Health Sciences Division, Oak Ridge Associated Universities, Oak Ridge, TN **[247]**

Michael J. Hill, Bacterial Metabolism Research Laboratory, Public Health Laboratory Service Center for Applied Microbiology and Research, Salisbury, UK **[263]**

The number in brackets is the opening page number of the contributor's article.

Gretchen L. Humason, Marmoset Research Program, Medical and Health Sciences Division, Oak Ridge Associated Universities, Oak Ridge, TN [247]

John G. Hunter, Division of Gastroenterology, Departments of Surgery and Medicine, University of Utah School of Medicine, Salt Lake City, UT [151]

Clarence C. Lushbaugh, Marmoset Research Program, Medical and Health Sciences Division, Oak Ridge Associated Universities, Oak Ridge, TN [247]

Arthur H. McArthur, Marmoset Research Program, Medical and Health Sciences Division, Oak Ridge Associated Universities, Oak Ridge, TN [247]

Douglas B. McGill, Division of Gastroenterology, Mayo Clinic, Rochester, MN [45]

Gail E. McKeown-Eyssen, Ludwig Institute for Cancer Research and Department of Preventive Medicine and Biostatistics, University of Toronto, Toronto, Ontario, Canada [277]

Norman D. Nigro, Department of Surgery, Wayne State University School of Medicine, Detroit, MI [161]

Masato Ohshima, Tumor Pathology and Pathogenesis Section, Laboratory of Comparative Carcinogenesis, Division of Cancer Etiology, National Cancer Institute, Frederick, MD [203]

Andrew B. Onderdonk, Infectious Diseases Research Laboratory, Tufts University School of Veterinary Medicine, Boston, MA [237]

Bandaru S. Reddy, Division of Nutrition and Endocrinology, Naylor Dana Institute for Disease Prevention, American Health Foundation, Valhalla, NY [285]

Robert H. Riddell, Department of Pathology, McMaster University Medical Center, Hamilton, Ontario, Canada [77]

Morton K. Schwartz, Department of Clinical Chemistry, Memorial Sloan-Kettering Cancer Center, New York, NY [57]

Roy G. Shorter, Department of Pathology and Medicine, Mayo Medical School, Rochester, MN [91]

Carol Smith, Department of Clinical Chemistry, Memorial Sloan-Kettering Cancer Center, New York, NY [57]

John A. Spratt, Department of Surgery, Duke University Hospital, Durham, NC [103]

John S. Spratt, Department of Surgery at the J. Graham Cancer Center, University of Louisville, Louisville, KY [103]

John R. Stroehlein, GI Section, Baylor College of Medicine, The Methodist Hospital, Houston, TX [121]

Jerrold M. Ward, Tumor Pathology and Pathogenesis Section, Laboratory of Comparative Carcinogenesis, Division of Cancer Etiology, National Cancer Institute, Frederick, MD [203]

Sidney J. Winawer, Department of Gastroenterology, Memorial Sloan-Kettering Cancer Center, New York, NY [57]

David P. Winchester, Department of Surgery, Northwestern University Medical School, Evanston Hospital, Evanston, IL [13]

Foreword

The symposium from which these papers stem was developed after enquiry about the most useful information, of practical worth, in the current and future attack on colorectal cancer. The premise was entertained that early detection, followed by earlier management, would allow more likelihood of cure, improved survival, and a better quality of life. Emphasis on curative management in advanced and end-stage cancer reflects poorly on our mission to control this disease. To redress this we sought to emphasize screening mechanisms and their applicability, to define risk (inherited and environmental), and to explore practical implications of current research.

Adenomas of the large bowel require much more attention as proximate risk factors for cancer. There is compelling evidence for this. References are well listed in this volume and emphasis is placed on the adenoma as a precursor to cancer; can they be prevented or destroyed early with resulting impact on the incidence of large bowel cancer? Diet, fiber, alcohol, and fat may have a protective or promoting role in cancer of the large bowel. The fiber story is well-known to all and has even permeated the food commercials—*but* do some fibers positively correlate with cancer?

Although genetic and environmental factors play a part in the genesis of large bowel cancer, it is a matter of balance between the two. There is a three-fold excess risk of developing large bowel cancer among relatives of a victim of the disease. We are in great need of biochemical markers to define these risks more accurately. The ensuing pages expand upon this area of research and its clinical applications.

The actual mechanisms of early detection and the newer methods of examination for fecal occult blood were introduced during the symposium as an exciting improvement in detection methods. The question remains—can we rely on patients' own interpretation of the improved tests? The use of laboratory animals has allowed study of carcinogenesis in the large bowel and we have to use caution in extrapolation of results to Homo sapiens.

Every effort must be made to reduce mortality from this disease. Much greater investment is needed on the proximate end of the cancer spectrum (i.e., prevention) than on the distal end—namely, treatment of the advanced disease. This may reduce the need for oncologists, which is an end in itself!

Once risk factors are defined, those who have them can be pursued in a totally asymptomatic population. There must be greater emphasis on primary, as well as secondary, prevention and only if the markers we seek become available, are we likely to have success in this arena.

Certain basic premises are examined in the use of screening tests—for example, those that pay for the test are more likely to complete it than those who receive it free. The verification of a positive test, including the subsequent diagnostic evaluation with its economic implications, has to be carefully appraised. The potential for screening to increase survival varies from 30% to 50%. This can have better impact than treating the established disease, but no study has proven that screening reduces mortality.

Those tests that are dependent on heme which can be reduced to porphyrins in the gastrointestinal tract, render the guaiac test negative, and it is of interest, for example, that the storing of fecal specimens allows degradation to porphyrins to occur. The Hemoccult test, the HemoQuant, Early Detector, and ColoScreen are all reviewed in this volume and dimensions of the challenge of early detection is well-stated by the different authors. Guidance is required on the indications for proctocolectomy, and as markers are developed this radical procedure may be better justified.

A singular feature of the text and the symposium is the interrelationship of the various authors to one another which conveys a sense of action in concert and an anticipation of better care to come. The sensitive issues of pathologically dictated radical surgery are examined and, without question, there is anticipation that the need for the latter—namely, radical surgery— may diminish; perhaps the colostomy will become obsolete.

Animal studies are providing fascinating pointers toward dietary induction of colorectal cancer. The metabolic products in the breakdown of carcinogenic agents are becoming better defined in their action, some of which are organ specific. Inhibition of tumorigenesis in the animal model has been successfully translated to man and validates continued exploration of the mechanism under laboratory control.

These proceedings explore the correlation merited between animal and human studies in tumorigenesis within the large bowel; the intensity of dose and relationship to size of lesion is a province under intense study. At the cellular level the structural unity of an adenoma appears much more stable than a carcinoma. The binding of a tumor promoter to cells of a dysplastic nature and the mechanism of disruption of intercellular organization as a feature of the transition to malignancy is well examined. In inflammatory conditions where the continued high level of cellular proliferation within the colitic bowel or, in like fashion, with increase in an adenomatous mass, the probability of error in D.N.A. synthesis and the emergence of cells with malignant behavior has much greater potential. The experimental models elucidating this are fascinating in their construction. Unquestionably, the laboratory studies vary, reflecting dosage of carcinogen and the animal used. The differences in each system are explored as, indeed, are the patterns of metastasis—and the validity of the adenoma-carcinoma sequence.

Ulcerative colitis remains uncertain of etiology and challenging in its persistence. The guinea pig model used to study this is providing insight into premalignant cellular change. In studies so far, the knowledge gained about initiating and maintaining factors in ulcerative colitis could provide answers to this baffling problem. In itself this would be a major benefit resulting from the study of cellular change in the development of cancer. The use of the marmoset in the study of ulcerative colitis and the strong genetic pointers in the various species—especially the colitis precursor stage—provide tremendous opportunity to manipulate the animal model and isolate factors which are difficult, if not impossible, to manage in humans.

The carcinogenicity of dietary meat or fat, and the protective action of dietary cereal fiber is well presented and the current status and problems with this research in groups of patients under study is well portrayed. Large bowel cancer is preventable and this should be cherished as a realistic goal. Whether dietary discipline can be shown to have major impact on those with a dominantly hereditary predisposition, and whether we can use compelling evidence from the laboratory and human studies to change dietary habits for the better are questions in our minds. Maybe the disease is inherently an outcome of human weakness and we face, on the basis of the presentations in this book, the sensitive questions of eugenics and discipline of nutrition, both of which are inherent features in the freedom of the individual.

Participants in this symposium are all leaders in their field and it is hoped that the observations contained in this volume will stimulate thought, new ideas, better management, and—above all—efforts toward the reduction of mortality from carcinoma of the large bowel.

John R.F. Ingall, M.D.
Anthony J. Mastromarino, Ph.D.

Acknowledgments

This document is the product of cooperation between the University of Texas (specifically, the National Large Bowel Cancer Project), Wayne State University (specifically, the Department of Surgery), with financial support from the American Cancer Society, Michigan Cancer Foundation, Warner Lambert Corporation, Pentax Precision Instrument Corporation, Pharmacia Laboratories, and SmithKline Diagnostics, Inc.

General Motors Corporation most graciously provided transportation for the social component of the conference held at the Detroit Institute of Arts. This occasion replenished the participants' intellect and gave sustenance for the second day.

One must also acknowledge the courtesy of the members of the Colorectal Board in their advice and, especially, Dr. Norman Nigro for his unflagging support of the program and concept.

The entire proceedings were reassembled and retyped by Mrs. Elizabeth Holben, to whom we are deeply indebted. It is hoped that the uniformity and standard of the type will add to the esthetic appearance of the text. Ms. Patricia Barrett and Mr. Jeffrey Mossoff of the Department of Surgery at Wayne State University, also played a major role in developing the conference; and Ms. Deborah Maloney of the National Large Bowel Cancer Project is seen as being invaluable as a coordinator between the two major institutions involved.

The vastness of the territory covered and the opportunity to introduce new concepts for the first time made the burden of organization lighter. For those who are not named in the foregoing, please accept that the co-editors of these proceedings are most appreciative of every gesture on their behalf.

Carcinoma of the Large Bowel and Its Precursors, pages 1–12
© 1985 Alan R. Liss, Inc.

OVERVIEW OF EPIDEMIOLOGY AND RISK FACTORS ASSOCIATED WITH
COLORECTAL CANCER

Jerome J. DeCosse, M.D., Ph.D., Chairman
Jean-Claude Bayle, M.D., Fellow

Department of Surgery
Memorial Sloan-Kettering Cancer Center
New York City, New York 10021

In what may be a bit over-simplified, the subject of risk factors for large bowel cancer in a westernized society can be brought into focus by the following statement: If 100 consecutive patients with large bowel cancer came to your office, probably one would have a background of familial polyposis, one a history of chronic active ulcerative colitis and approximately 13 would have a family history of large bowel cancer suggestive of a genetic linkage. Most, but not all of these 13 patients would have a few adenomas scattered throughout the large bowel. Among the remaining 85 patients who have "sporadic" large bowel cancer, approximately 20 also would have one or a few large bowel adenomas.

Behind this display of histopathologic risk factors are the expressions of both genetic and environmental events presumed important in induction of large bowel neoplasia. As a working hypothesis, the biological consequences of these genetic, or initiating, events interact with subsequent environmentally-generated, or promotional, events to result in adenomas and later large bowel cancer. In this context, cancer in familial polyposis, which must be the consequence of a powerful genetic mutation, still requires environmental influences in a setting of biological amplification from the genetic mutation.

The environment of the large bowel mucosa is the content of the gut lumen. Here it is hypothesized that exogenously-derived sterols, particularly fat, and endogenously-circulating sterols, mainly bile salts and acids, are degraded by colonic microflora to produce carcinogens such as deoxycholic acid, lithocholic acid, and other metabolites to which the mucosal cells of the large bowel are exposed. It is these environmental, or promotional events that are thought to explain racial and geographic differences in both the incidence and distribution of adenomas and large bowel cancer. It is also these promotional events that provide the basis for the "fat and fiber hypotheses" for induction of large bowel neoplasia and for initial efforts to inhibit the development of large bowel adenomas and cancer.

PROXIMATE RISK FACTORS

Adenomas of the large bowel deserve more attention as proximate risk factors. From an epidemiologic point of view, the association between adenomas and large bowel cancer is supported by several lines of evidence. The incidence of large bowel cancer closely parallels the prevalence of adenomatous polyps in all populations so far studied. White, blacks, and orientals have a low prevalence if they migrate to areas of high large bowel cancer risk. The difference in the prevalence of adenomas between migrant and native Japanese is consistent with the incidence of large bowel cancer in the two groups. In the populations studied, the risk of large bowel cancer increases with the size and multiplicity of adenomas, thus suggesting a dose-response relationship. For a thoughtful, recently published review of this subject, a short text edited by Correa and Haenszel (1982) is recommended.

For these reasons and other evidence from histopathology, most informed pathologists conclude that all, or almost all, large bowel cancers emerge from large bowel adenomas. An extension of this view is that the epidemiology of large bowel cancer can be studied as the epidemiology of large bowel adenomas. A still further extension is that the prevention or destruction of large bowel adenomas will reduce the incidence of large bowel cancer. There is evidence to support this view (Dales et al 1974; Gilbertsen 1974) and other trials are currently underway.

GEOGRAPHIC EPIDEMIOLOGY

The geographic differences in the incidence of large bowel cancer are well known, with the higher incidence in urbanized, westernized, affluent societies. It appears that these differences, and differences in risk related to social class, occupation and religion may be explained by differences in diet. Alcohol consumption, particularly beer, may be relevant for rectal cancer (Pollack et al 1984). Differences in diet may provide the best correlation with differences in the incidence of large bowel cancer. The strongest positive correlations with large bowel cancer are with animal protein and total fat intake. The strongest negative correlations with large bowel cancer are with an increased intake of cereals, legumes and nuts, suggesting the importance of fiber (Bjelke 1974; Armstrong and Doll 1975; Howell 1975; Correa and Haenszel 1982).

Of all dietary changes studied in humans thus far, an increase in grain fiber probably has the best association with the reduction in carcinogenesis. In case control studies (Modan et al 1975) and population studies (Jensen and MacLennan 1979), fiber protected against large bowel cancer. In the studies of Irving and Drasar (1973) only cereal fiber was inversely related to large bowel carcinogenesis, whereas fruit fiber was positively correlated with cancer.

Geographic epidemiology has also provided information to suggest that differences exist between the rectum and colon in the etiology of large bowel cancer (Correa and Haenszel 1982). In the low risk population (Cali) the incidence of cancer is distributed much more uniformly throughout the large bowel. In the high risk population, however, there is a much greater proportion of cancer immediately cephalad or proximate to the mid-rectum with a particular emphasis in the segment between 6 to 15 cm above the anus.

In a study of polyposis patients, we found that the distal 5 cm of rectum was relatively spared of large bowel adenomas when compared with the more cephalad 10 cm of rectum. Hence, in this genetically-driven inherited disease there appears to be a nonrandom distribution of adenomas in the rectum. It appears there may be a difference between the traditional anatomical definition of the rectum and the functional definition with respect to large bowel neoplasia. Since there is no known difference in the histopathology of neoplasia of cancer within the large bowel, these differences may reflect differences in distribution of carcinogens within the gut lumen.

GENETIC EPIDEMIOLOGY

Aside from familial polyposis, a well known autosomal dominant disorder leading almost inexorably to adenomas and subsequently to large bowel cancer if untreated, genetic linkage is less striking in most patients with large bowel cancer. Although there are well known racial differences in incidence, race of itself does not seem unequivocally to affect the incidence of large bowel cancer - the difference observed can be explained alternatively by differences in environment and differences in recording of health care.

Hence, only a minor fraction of patients with large bowel cancer can be linked by familial aggregation. However, a three-fold excess risk for large bowel cancer exists among relatives of a patient with this malignancy (Woolf 1958: Macklin 1960; Lovett 1976). Excluding polyposis, genetic risk factors are difficult to ascertain; there is a need for quantifiable biochemical markers that will identify the high risk patient. Ornithine decarboxylase is an interesting candidate (Luk and Baylin 1984; Rozhin et al 1984).

There does appear to be a sex-related difference in the incidence of large bowel cancer. Most, but not all studies show a male excess of rectal cancer. There may be a decrease in the mortality from large bowel cancer in women, but not in men. There are other sex differences in incidence by geographic area, age, anatomic location and time periods. Increasing parity may decrease the risk of colon cancer, especially right-sided colon cancer (Potter and McMichael 1983). Large bowel cancer in women is associated with an increased risk for breast and endometrial cancer. Are there subtle endocrine relationships in large bowel cancer in woman or are these differences explained entirely by differences in diet?

It is also apparent that familial polyposis is a systemic disturbance in growth regulation. Our investigations of a group of polyposis patients have demonstrated that other systemic defects exist or the gene for these systemic defects may be presumed present in virtually every affected patient. A variety of biological in vitro studies show that fibroblasts are regularly abnormal in polyposis patients whether or not extracolonic manifestations are present. These findings argue against separating familial polyposis from Gardner's syndrome; one term should be used.

METABOLIC EPIDEMIOLOGY

Epidemiological data suggest that secondary bile acids have a role in the pathogenesis of large bowel cancer. Fecal specimens from subjects living in industrialized countries which have a high incidence of large bowel cancer contain higher concentrations of secondary bile acids than specimens from African or Asian nations where there is a low incidence of large bowel cancer (Drasar and Irving 1973; Wynder and Reddy 1974). Similarly, fecal concentrations of secondary bile acids are higher in patients with large bowel cancer than in controls (Hill 1975; Hill et al 1975; Reddy and Wynder 1977). It has also been observed that secondary bile acids act as cocarcinogens in experimentally-induced large bowel cancer in laboratory animals (Narisawa et al 1974; Reddy et al 1976a and 1977).

The carcinogens responsible for initiating and promoting human large bowel cancer have not been identified but the amount of dietary fat is thought to determine the concentration of secondary bile acids. Bile acids, and their products, are thought to act as tumor promotors and to alter intestinal epithelial microsomal enzyme systems whose functions probably include activation and deactivation of carcinogens. The protective effect of certain dietary fibers may be dilutional or may involve metabolism of carcinogens, cocarcinogens or promoters. In addition, studies of fecal mutagens suggest that metabolites of bacteria, particularly mutagenic ether-lipids called fecapentaenes, may be important in the induction of large bowel cancer (Gupta et al 1984).

EXTENSION OF EPIDEMIOLOGIC OBSERVATION TO LABORATORY
INVESTIGATION

The issues of fat and fiber in large bowel cancer were
addressed at length in the volume, "Diet, Nutrition and
Cancer" (1982). The conclusion from this review was that
specific components of fiber, rather than total dietary
fiber, are likely to be responsible for any protective
benefit that is achieved.

We have reviewed the literature pertinent to
experimentally-induced large bowel cancer and use of fiber
and fat. We found it difficult to scrutinize these papers
because of possible confounding variables such as variations in species, sex, and age of the experimental animals:
type, dosage, and duration of carcinogens; the exact histopathology of the tumors that occurred (Ward et al 1973a;
Ward 1974; Pazharisski 1975; Maskens 1976; Maskens and
Dujardin-Loits 1981; Shamsuddin and Trump 1981): kind,
amount, and mode of administration of fiber: and ancillary
confounding variables such as the use or non-use of bedding
which itself contains fiber and is assimilated by the
experimental animals (Wise and Gilburt 1980).

We reviewed 18 studies of insoluble fiber in 17
publications. All used the rat as the experimental model
and dimethylhydrazine (DMH) or azoxymethane (AOM) as the
carcinogen. Carcinogenesis was inhibited by wheat bran in
7 of 9 studies, by nonspecified insoluble fiber in 1 of 2,
by cellulose in 5 of 6, and by hemicellulose in 1 study.
Hence, protection against large bowel carcinogenesis was
found in 14 of 18 experiments.

Among the remaining 4 studies, there was concern about
the experimental design of each. In one experiment, wheat
fiber was administered for only 15 weeks during a total
experimental period of 24 to 25 weeks (Bauer et al 1979).
In another, the proportion of rats developing a tumor (3 of
12 on the control diet and 4 of 12 on wheat fiber) was the
least of all studies examined (Jacobs 1983). In the negative study with a nonspecified bran, results were based on
analysis one year after the initial DMH injection (Cruse et
al 1978); if the data are analyzed within the same window
as other publications a protective effect is noted. In the
fourth negative study which applied cellulose (Ward et al
1973b), the weekly dose of AOM was approximately twice the

amount of AOM administered in another study where cellulose was protective (Nigro et al 1979).

The inference from this scrutiny is that the insoluble components of fiber provided some protection against experimental large bowel carcinogenesis. In contrast, soluble fibers such as pectin had no value in 3 of 4 experiments (Bauer et al 1979 and 1981; Freeman et al 1980). In the experiment where pectin had a protective effect (Watanabe et al 1979), the rats fed the diet containing pectin showed about 25% less body weight compared with those fed the control diet.

The role of fat was also evaluated. Among 10 publications examined, comparing a diet enriched in fat versus a control diet, an enhancing effect of fat was noted in 9. When the negative study was compared to the others, two major differences were found - a very low dose of DMH and a very long interval to examination, the animals being sacrificed up to 60 weeks following the initial injection of carcinogen (Nauss et al 1983).

In 11 publications, polyunsaturated fats were compared to saturated fats. Polyunsaturated fats had a greater enhancing effect in 6, a lesser effect in 3, and there was no difference in 2. Where saturated fats were noted to have more of an enhancing effect, differences in other dietary supplements may have accounted for this discrepancy. In one study, soybean proteins were added to the corn oil, and beef proteins to the beef fat (Reddy et al 1976b), and it has been demonstrated that mutagenic compounds exist in beef extract. One of them, 2-amino-3-methylimidazo (4,5-f) quinoline (IQ), has been shown to induce colon carcinoma in the rat (Takayama et al 1984). In the second experiment, lipotropes were added to the saturated fat (Rogers and Newberne 1973), whereas in a similar experiment, without lipotropes, the enhancing effect of polyunsaturated fat was more pronounced (Rogers and Newberne 1975). In the third study, the polyunsaturated fat was partially hydrogenated (Rogers et al 1980). In the two studies without differences noted, when fats were used alone (Wilson et al 1977; Trudel et al 1983), the addition of insoluble fiber to the diet was more protective on saturated fats than on polyunsaturated fats.

The inferences of this analysis of fat are that fat has an enhancing effect on the induction of neoplasma of the colon in the experimental animals, and that this effect is generally more pronounced for polyunsaturated than for saturated fats.

INTERVENTIONAL EPIDEMIOLOGY

These epidemiologic, histopathologic and biochemical risk factors have lead to intervention in human large bowel carcinogenesis. These will be developed at greater length within this volume. These interventions include screening and the quest for better methods to identify high risk patients, the identification and removal of large bowel adenomas, and the utility of cytologic dysplasia as a risk factor in chronic ulcerative colitis.

It is also these data that have led to strategies for biochemical and dietary interventions which already show exciting potential for the future. As a final generalization, we submit there is sufficient evidence of both value and safety to recommend to the public that a diet low in fat, high in insoluble fiber and vitamin-enriched will protect against the development of large bowel adenomas and cancer.

REFERENCES

Armstrong B, Doll R (1975). Environmental factors and cancer incidence and mortality in different countries with special reference to dietary practices. Int J Cancer 15:617.
Bauer HG, Asp N-G, Oste R, Dahlqvist A, Fredlund PE (1979). Effect of dietary fiber on the induction of colorectal tumors and fecal β-glucuronidase activity in the rat. Cancer Res 39:3752.
Bauer HG, Asp N-G, Dahlqvist A, Fredlund PE, Nyman M, Oste R (1981). Effect of two kinds of pectin and guar gum on 1,2-dimethylhydrazine initiation of colon tumors and on fecal β-glucuronidase activity in the rat. Cancer Res 41:2518.
Bjelke E (1974). Epidemiologic studies of cancer of the stomach, colon, and rectum; with special emphasis on the role of diet. Scand J Gastroenterol. 9(31):1.
Committee on Diet, Nutrition and Cancer, National Research Council (1982) "Diet, Nutrition, and Cancer." Washington: National Academy Press.

Correa P, Haenszel W (1982). Epidemiology of Cancer of the Digestive Tract. Boston: Martinus Nishoff, p 85.

Cruse JP, Lewin MR, Clark CG (1978). Failure of bran to protect against experimental colon cancer in rats. Lancet 2:1278.

Dales LG, Friedman GD, Collen MF (1974). Evaluation of a periodic multiphasic health checkup. Methods Inf Med 13:140.

Draser BS, Irving D (1973). Environmental factors and cancer of the colon and breast. Br J Cancer 27:167.

Freeman HJ, Spiller GA, Kim YS (1980). A double-blind study on the effects of differing purified cellulose and pectin fibre diets on 1,2-dimethylhydrazine-induced rat colonic neoplasia. Cancer Res 40:2661.

Gilbertsen VA (1974). Proctosigmoidoscopy and polypectomy in reducing the incidence of rectal cancer. Cancer 34:936.

Gupta I, Suzuki, Bruce WR, Krepinsky JJ, Yates P (1984). A model study of fecapentaenes: mutagens of bacterial origin with alkylating properties. Science 225:521.

Hill MJ (1975). The role of colon anaerobes in the metabolism of bile acids and steroids, and its relation to colon cancer. Cancer 36:2387.

Hill MJ, Drasar BS, Williams REO, Meade TW, Cox AG, Simpson JEP, Morson BC (1975). Fecal bile-acids and clostridia in patients with cancer of the large bowel. Lancet 1:535.

Howell MA (1975). Diet as an etiological factor in the development of cancers of the colon and rectum. J Chronic Dis 28:67.

Irving D, Drasar BS 1973). Fibre and cancer of the colon. Br J Cancer 28:462.

Jacobs LR (1983). Enhancement of rat colon carcinogenesis by wheat bran consumption during the stage of 1,2-dimethylhydrazine administration. Cancer Res 43:4057.

Jensen OM, MacLennan R (1979). Dietary factors and colorectal cancer in Scandinavia. Isr J Med Sci 15:329.

Lovett E (1976). Family studies in cancer of the colon and rectum. Br J Surg 63:13.

Luk GD, Baylin SB (1984). Ornithine decarboxylase as a biological marker in familial colonic polyposis. N Eng J Med 311:80.

Macklin MT (1960). Inheritance of cancer of the stomach and large intestine in man. J Natl Cancer Inst 24:551.

Maskens AP (1976). Histogenesis and growth pattern of 1,2-dimethylhydrazine-induced rat colon adenocarcinoma. Cancer Res 36:1585.

Maskens AP, Dujardin-Loits R-M (1981). Experimental adenomas and carcinomas of the large intestine behave as distinct entities: most carcinomas arise de novo in flat mucosa. Cancer 47:81.

Modan B, Barell BA, Lubin F, Modan M, Greenberg RA, Graham S (1975). Low-fiber intake as an etiologic factor in cancer of the colon. J Natl Cancer Inst 55:15.

Narisawa T, Magadia NE, Weisburger JH, Synder EL (1974). Promoting effect of bile acids in colon carcinogenesis after intrarectal installation of N-methyl-N'-nitro N-nitrosoquanidine in rats. J Natl Cancer Inst 53:1093.

Nauss KM, Locniskar M, Newberne PM (1983). Effect of alterations in the quality and quantity of dietary fat on 1,2-dimethylhydrazine-induced colon tumorigenesis in rats. Cancer Res 43:4083.

Nigro ND, Bull AW, Klopfer BA, Pak MS, Campbell RL (1979). Effect of dietary fiber on azoxymethane-induced intestinal carcinogenesis in rats. J Natl Cancer Inst 62:1097.

Pollack ES, Nomura AM, Heilbrun LK, Stemmermann GN, Green SB (1984). Prospective study of alcohol consumption and cancer. N Engl J Med 310:617.

Potter JD, McMichael AJ (1983). Large Bowel cancer in women in relation to reproductive and hormonal factors: a case control study. JNCI 71:703.

Pozharisski KM (1975). Morphology and morphogenesis of experimental epithelial tumors of the intestine. J Natl Cancer Inst 54:1115.

Reddy BS, Narasawa T, Weisburger JH, Wynder EL (1976a). Brief communication: promoting effect of sodium deoxycholate on colon adenocarcinomas in germ-free rats. J Natl Cancer Inst 56:441.

Reddy BS, Narisawa T, Weisburger JH (1976b). Effect of a diet with high levels of protein and fat on colon carcinogenesis in F344 rats treated with 1,2-dimethylhydrazine. J Natl Cancer Inst 57:567.

Reddy BS, Watanabe K, Weisburger JH, Wynder EL (1977). Promoting effect of bile acids in colon carcinogenesis in germ-free and conventional F344 rats. Cancer Res 37:3238.

Reddy BS, Wynder EL (1977). Metabolic epidemiology of colon cancer. Fecal bile acids and neutral sterols in colon cancer patients and patients with adenomatous polyps. Cancer 39:2533.

Rogers AE, Newberne PM (1973). Dietary enhancement of intestinal carcinogenesis by dimethylhydrazine in rats. Nature 246:491.

Rogers AE, Newberne PM (1975). Dietary effects on chemical carcinogenesis in animal models for colon and liver tumors. Cancer Res 35:3427.

Rogers AE, Lenhart G, Morrison G (1980). Influence of dietary lipotrope and lipid content on aflatoxin B_1, N-2-fluorenylacetamide, and 1,2-dimethylhydrazine carcinogenesis in rats. Cancer Res 40:2802.

Rozhin J, Wilson PS, Bull AW, Nigro ND (1984). Ornithine decarboxylase activity in the rat and human colon. Cancer Res 44:3226.

Shamsuddin AKM, Trump BF (1981). Colon epithelium. II. In vivo studies of colon carcinogenesis. Light microscopic, histochemical, and ultrastructural studies of histogenesis of azoxymethane-induced colon carcinomas in Fischer 344 rats. JNCI 66:389.

Takayama S, Nakatsuru Y, Masuda M, Ohgaki H, Sato S, Sugimura T (1984). Demonstration of carcinogenicity in F344 rate of 2-amino-3-methyl-imidazo (4,5-f) quinoline from broiled sardine, fried beef and beef extract. Gann 75:467.

Trudel JL, Senterman MK, Brown RA (1983). The fat/fiber antagonism in experimental colon carcinogenesis. Surgery 94:691.

Ward JM, Yamamoto RS, Brown CA (1973a). Pathology of intestinal neoplasms and other lesions in rats exposed to azoxymethane. J Natl Cancer Inst 51:1029.

Ward JM, Yamamoto RS, Weisburger JH (1973b). Brief communication: cellulose dietary bulk and axoxymethane-induced intestinal cancer. J Natl Cancer Inst 51:713.

Ward JM (1974). Morphogenesis of chemically induced neoplasms of the colon and small intestine in rats. Lab Invest 30:505.

Watanabe K, Reddy BS, Weisburger JH, Kritchevsky D (1979). Effect of dietary alfalfa, pectin, and wheat bran on azoxymethane- or methylnitrosourea-induced colon carcinogenesis in F344 rats. J Natl Cancer Inst 63:141.

Wilson RB, Hutcheson DP, Wideman L (1977). Dimethylhydrazine-induced colon tumors in rats fed diets containing beef fat or corn oil with and without wheat bran. Am J Clin Nutr 30:176.

Wise A, Gilburt DJ (1980). The variability of dietary fibre in laboratory animal diets and its relevance to the control of experimental conditions. Food Cosmet Toxicol 18:643.

Woolf CM (1958). A genetic study of carcinoma of the large intestine. Amer J Hum Genet 10:42.

Wynder EL, Reddy BS (1974). Metabolic epidemiology of colorectal cancer. Cancer 34:801.

Carcinoma of the Large Bowel and Its Precursors, pages 13–21

SCREENING FOR COLORECTAL NEOPLASIA

David P. Winchester, M.D.
Northwestern University Medical School
Chief, Surgical Oncology
Evanston Hospital
Evanston, Illinois 60201

INTRODUCTION

Until primary prevention of colorectal cancer is possible, efforts must continue in secondary prevention (early detection) as a means of reducing mortality from the disease. Ideally, secondary prevention should consist of detection of pathologically early-stage, asymptomatic colorectal tumors in a cost effective, reasonably safe manner and with a significantly demonstrable reduction in mortality.

A common source of confusion is the difference between screenig and diagnosis of disease. Screening refers to the search for disease in a presumably asymptomatic population while diagnosis is the outcome of a test or tests applied to a population in whom disease is suspected on the basis of results of screening or symptoms.

The American Cancer Society in their "Guidelines for the Cancer-Related Checkup" (Eddy 1980) stated that, in making recommendations, there were four concerns: one, there must be good evidence that each test or procedure recommended is medically effective in reducing morbidity or mortality; two, the medical benefits must outweigh the risks; three, the cost of each test or procedure must be reasonable compared to its expected benefits; four, the recommended actions must be practical and feasible.

SCREENING COMPONENTS

Screening for colorectal neoplasia begins with a thoughtful history for symptoms to assure that one is dealing with an asymptomatic patient, and an inquiry about risk factors. Common risk factors include a personal or family history of colorectal neoplasia, chronic ulcerative colitis, and familial polyposis. Individuals falling into any of these categories should not be considered for screening as in an asymptomatic population, but should be put into more intense surveillance protocols.

The remaining components to be regarded as screening tests include digital rectal examination, proctosigmoidoscopy and the stool guaiac test.

DIGITAL RECTAL EXAMINATION

Digital rectal examination has long been regarded as a simple, safe and cost effective method of detecting abnormalities of the rectum and prostate gland. The potential risks seem small and include a false sense of security and needless workup for a false positive result.

Because of these factors, no one has found it necessary to subject this screening examination to rigorous scientific investigation. One trial conducted by the KAISER FOUNDATION HEALTH PLAN, involving approximately 5,000 individuals, demonstrated a decreased mortality from colorectal cancer in a group screened with digital rectal examination, blood studies for anemia and sigmoidoscopy versus an unscreened population (Dales 1979). It is possible that digital rectal examination played an important role in this study.

PROCTOSIGMOIDOSCOPY

Although the results of three studies support the use of proctosigmoidoscopy, this test has been grossly under-utilized by both the public and the profession. Many factors account for its disfavor including cost, inconvenience, discomfort and low motivation.

The previously mentioned Kaiser study (Dales 1979)

included sigmoidoscopy as one of the screening tests. The observed decrease in mortality undoubtedly was due in part to sigmoidoscopy, which was performed in approximately one-third of the group.

A second study, conducted by the University of Minnesota over a long period of time, involving over 18,000 patients (Gilbertsen 1974) achieved an 85% reduction in the expected number of cases of rectal cancer by a routine policy of sigmoidoscopic polypectomy.

The third study was coordinated by the Strang Clinic in New York (Hertz 1960). Twenty-six thousand, one hundred and twenty six individuals over the age of 45 were offered sigmoidoscopy annually over an 18-year period. Cancer was found in 58 patients and a long term survival rate after treatment was nearly 90%, far in excess of survival rates observed in unscreened populations.

Flexible fiberoptic technology has expanded the scope of the examination with less discomfort. The two instruments in this category which are useful for screening are the 35 cm and 60 cm flexible scopes. Several investigators (Christie 1980; Crespi 1978; Winnan 1980) report a gain in diagnostic yield of 100% or more compared to rigid proctoscopy using the 60 cm flexible scope rather than the rigid 25 cm proctoscope. Marks (Marks 1979) and his colleagues reported similar favorable results. The flexible scope attained an average depth of 55 cm compared with 20 cm with the rigid scope. The average time to perform the 60 cm flexible exam was 9.4 minutes compared with 5.9 minutes with the rigid scope.

Although flexible scopes are more comfortable for the patient and have a higher yield, the problems of cost and adequate training for examiners remain. McCray (McCray 1981) observed that an average of 50 procedures under supervision were required for training physicians and one out of five could never attain adequate skills.

Recently, 30 and 35 cm flexible scopes have been under investigation for screening asymptomatic patients (Winawer 1982; Ufberg 1982; Weissman 1982). Apparently nonendoscopists can be much more readily trained with these instruments than with the 60 cm scope. Six examinations or fewer were required for training. The average examination time was 5.3 minutes and the patients reported little or no discomfort.

THE STOOL BLOOD TEST

Early attempts to chemically identify blood in the stool were unsuccessful because the methods utilized resulted in an unacceptably high false positive rate. In 1971 Greegor (Greegor 1971) reported the use of impregnated guaiac slides over a three day period to detect occult blood. Since then this method has gained widespread acceptance and several other products are on the market.

The chemical basis for the test is the phenolic oxidation of guaiac to a blue compound which is catalyzed by a peroxidase-like enzyme of hemoglobin. Several factors are responsible for the test result, including storage time, rehydration (which increases the number of positive tests), consumption of foods high in peroxidase-like content, such as broccoli and turnips, and the site and rate of bleeding from polyps and tumors (Gnauck 1984). Vitamin C may produce a falsely negative result, while iron ingestion may produce a false positive result. In general, the rate of positive slides has been low (2 - 5%); the false positive rate likewise low (1 - 2%); the predictive value for neoplasia, high (30 - 50%); and the pathologic stage earlier in screened populations (Winawer 1984).

The stool blood test is an attractive option for colorectal neoplasia screening because it is relatively cheap, can be easily marketed and seems to have a high degree of acceptance by both the profession and the public. Several reports indicate that it is effective in identifying pathologically earlier colorectal neoplasms, but a reduction in mortality has yet to be demonstrated. The false negative rate for colon cancer has been reported as low as approximately 8% (Roth 1982) and as high as 31% (Macrae 1982). Unfortunately adenomas bleed much less frequently and a false negative rate as high as 70% has been reported (Winawer 1980).

In 1978 a large scale study involving 54,000 individuals in the Chicago area was conducted and coordinated by the Illinois Division of the American Cancer Society in cooperation with the television medium (Winchester 1980). Early case finding was evident with 27 of 30 cancers found being modified Dukes A or B lesions. It was interesting that individuals who received free test slides were less apt to complete the test than those who paid a nominal fee. Nonetheless public motivation to complete the test was low. Of the 54,000 individuals requesting the test only 26% completed the series. Misinterpretation of test results was a potential problem identified. Diagnostic evaluation of screenees with positive test results by physicians was quite varied and often incomplete.

In 1983 a similar program was initiated to extend the observations of the 1978 study, more precisely define public attitudes about colon cancer and the stool blood test and to improve the existing guidelines for the test's use in community-based screening programs (Winchester 1983). A total of 106,551 individuals ordered Hemoccult II$^{(R)}$ kits and 45,658 or 43% properly completed and returned the kit. Five hundred and ninety-one (1.3%) were positive and, through diligent follow-up with the screen-ees , 85% reported seeing their physician. Diagnostic evaluation was again found to be variable and often incom-plete. Colorectal cancer was identified in 22 of 508 patients who could be evaluated (4.3%). Sixty-eight percent of this group had modified Dukes A or B lesions, confirming the value once again of early case finding. Polyps were discovered in 53 of the patients (10.4%). Sixty-seven percent of positive screenees were found to be positive on only one of three days tested, highlighting the importance of not repeating the stool blood test for a positive result but instead proceeding with appropriate diagnostic evaluation.

COST EFFECTIVENESS OF COLORECTAL CANCER SCREENING

Eddy analyzed the cost effectiveness of colorectal cancer screening and reported at the Third International Symposium on Colorectal Cancer. He utilized a computer model consisting of a set of mathematical equations describing the relationships between the important factors that affect the outcome of a colorectal cancer screening program. Key questions were posed to the attendees at that conference in various areas of expertise and the

results compiled as follows:
1. 90% of colorectal cancers arise from adenomatous polyps.
2. A precancerous adenoma is potentially detectable by sigmoidoscopy for seven years before it becomes invasive (range 0 - 14 years)
3. 44% of precancerous adenomas bleed prior to invasion (and are potentially detectable by the stool blood test.
4. For adenomas that do not bleed prior to invasion, bleeding begins an average of 2.5 years prior to invasion (range 0 - 6 years).
5. 30% of precancerous adenomas and cancers arise within practical reach of the rigid sigmoidoscope.
6. 50% of precancerous adenomas and cancers arise within practical reach of the flexible sigmoidoscope.
7. The random false negative rate of the stool blood test is 45%.
8. The random false negative rate of the sigmoidoscope is 20%.
9. The false positive rate of the stool blood test is 1.5%.
10. In the absence of screening it takes an average of two years for an invasive cancer to progress through local to regional disease, and one year to progress through regional to distant disease.
11. A stool blood test costs about $5, a rigid sigmoidoscopy costs $40, a flexible sigmoidoscopy costs $65, a workup of a patient with a positive stool blood test costs $820 (Eddy 1983).

Using this as a data base, the following questions and answers were developed:
1. What proportion of invasive cancers can be prevented by finding and removing adenomatous polyps with an annual stool blood test? About 15%. With an annual stool blood test and a rigid sigmoidoscopy every three years? About 25%.
2. How much will screening change long-term survival? Screening will increase the chance of a colorectal cancer patient not dying of disease by about 30 - 50%, depending on the screening strategy.

3. How much will mortality be decreased? By about 1/3 (20 - 40%, depending on the strategy).
4. How long will screening prolong a patient's expected lifetime? With screening, the life expectancy of a colorectal cancer patient is increased by about 2 to 2.5 years, depending on the strategy.
5. How much will it cost and what are the risks? The lifetime costs vary from less than $100 to about $700 depending on the strategy; the main risk is from the workup of a false positive stool blood test, if a person is screened annually with a stool blood test from age 50 to 75, he or she will have about a one in four chance of eventually needing a workup.
6. In terms of cost and resources, how does screening for colorectal cancer compare with other medical activities? Considering the increase in life expectancy and the financial costs, screening for colorectal cancer appears to be a quite effective and efficient use of resources compared with other medical activities, delivering a person/year of life in a large population for about $1000.
7. What tests should be used? Compared to annual tests with both the stool blood test and rigid sigmoidoscopy, an annual stool blood test alone delivers about 2/3 of the effectiveness at about 1/6 the cost; using a flexible sigmoidoscope rather than a rigid sigmoidoscope increases the benefit by about 25%, at an increase in cost of about 50%.
8. At what age? Compared with screening with an annual stool blood test from age 50 to 75, beginning screening at age 41 increases the benefit by about 17%, at about twice the cost.
9. At what frequency? Compared with an annual stool blood test, a biannual stool blood test delivers about 2/3 of the benefit at about 40% of the cost; compared with an annual stool blood test and an annual sigmoidoscopy, changing the frequency of sigmoidoscopies to every three years decreases the benefit by about 10%, while decreasing the cost by about 50%.
10. Is screening worth the effort? These estimates do not directly answer the question as to whether

screening for colorectal cancer is worthwhile nor do they identify the "optimum" strategy or tell which screening age or frequence of choice of tests is the "best"; in the end, these are value judgements requiring comparison of the potential benefits of different strategies with the costs and risks: the purpose of this analysis was to provide practicing physicians and health planners with some of the information needed to make these comparisons (Eddy 1983).

RECOMMENDATIONS

Based on the data which have been presented, the American Cancer Society recommends that all persons age 40 and over should have a digital rectal examination annually; a stool guaiac slide test should be added at age 50 on an annual basis and sigmoidoscopy should be performed every three to five years after two initial negative sigmoidoscopies one year apart.

REFERENCES

Christie JP (1980). Flexible sigmoidoscopy: why, where, and when? Am J Gastroenterol 73:70-72.

Crespi M, Casale V, Grassi A (1978). Flexible sigmoidoscopy: a potential advance in cancer control. Gastrointest Endosc 24:291-292.

Dales LG, Friedman GD, Collen MF (1979). Evaluating periodic multiphasic health checkups: a controlled trial. J Chronic Dis 32:385-404.

Eddy D (1980). Guidelines for the cancer-related checkup: recommendations and rationale. CA 30:194-240.

Eddy D (1983). Proceedings of the Third International Symposium on Colorectal Cancer.

Gilbertsen VA (1974). Proctosigmoidoscopy and polypectomy in reducing the incidence of rectal cancer. Cancer 34: 936-939.

Gnauck R, Macrae FA, Fleisher M (1984). How to perform the fecal occult blood test. CA 34:134-147.

Greegor DH (1971). Occult blood testing for detection of asymptomatic colon cancer. Cancer 28:131-134.

Hertz RE, Deddish MR, Day E (1960). Value of periodic examination in detecting cancer of the rectum and colon. Postgrad Med 27:290-294.

Macrae FA, St John DJ (1982). Relationship between patterns of bleeding and Hemoccult sensitivity in patients with colorectal cancers or adenomas. Gastroenterology 82:891-898.

Marks G, Boggs W, Castro AF, Gathright JB, Ray JE, Salvati E (1979). Sigmoidoscopic examinations with rigid and flexible fiberoptic sigmoidoscopes in the surgeon's office. A comparative prospective study of effectiveness in 1,012 cases. Dis Colon Rectum 22:162-168.

McCray RS (1981). A fiberoptic sigmoidoscopy training program for cancer screening physicians. Gastrointest Endosc 27:137.

Roth A (1982). The results of Hemoccult test in 200 patients with gastrointestinal cancer, abstract #1303. Stockholm, World Congress of Gastroenterology.

Ufberg MH (1982). The 30 cm flexible sigmoidoscope-- preliminary experiemce. Pract Gastroenterol 6:35-36.

Weissman GS, Winawer SJ, Sergi M, Baldwin M, Miller C, Cummins R, Ephraim R, Ptak T, Talbott TM, Dixon JA, Schapiro M (1982). Preliminary results of a multicenter evaluation of a 30 cm flexible sigmoidoscope by nonendoscopists. Gastrointest Endosc 28:150.

Winawer SJ, Andrews M, Flehinger B (1980). Progress report on controlled trial of fecal occult blood testing for the detection of colorectal neoplasia. Cancer 45: 2959-2964.

Winawer SJ, Cummins R, Baldwin MP, Ptak A (1982). A new flexible sigmoidoscope for the generalist. Gastrointest Endosc 28:233-236.

Winawer SJ (1984). Introduction to position papers from the Third International Symposium on Colorectal Cancer. CA 34:130-133.

Winchester DP, Schull JH, Scanlon EF, Murrell JV, Smeltzer C, Vrba P, Iden M, Streelman DH, Magpayo R, Dow JW, Sylvester J (1980). A mass screening program for colorectal cancer using chemical testing for occult blood in the stool. Cancer 45:2955-2958.

Winchester DP, Sylvester J, Maher ML (1983). Risks and benefits of mass screening for colorectal neoplasia with the stool guaiac test. CA 33:333-343.

Winnan G. Berci G, Panish J. Talbat TM, Overhold BF, Mc-Callum RW (1980). Superiority of the flexible to the rigid sigmoidoscopoe in routine proctosigmoidoscopy. N Engl J Med 302:1011-1012.

Carcinoma of the Large Bowel and Its Precursors, pages 23–43
© 1985 Alan R. Liss, Inc.

PREMALIGNANT LESIONS OF THE COLORECTUM

Cecilia M. Fenoglio, M.D.
Chief, Laboratory Service (113)
Veterans Administration Medical Center
Albuquerque, New Mexico 87108

In the United States and other countries where diets high in fats, cholesterol and fried foods and low in fiber are consumed, colorectal carcinoma continues to be one of the most frequently encountered cancers in both males and females. Currently, it is responsible for about 126,000 newly diagnosed cancer patients in the United States. Therefore, the cure of colorectal cancer depends on identifying those patients who are at high risk for developing the disease, as well as identifying tissue changes that herald early preneoplastic events before they become capable of killing the patient. Fortunately, the usual developmental sequence involved in the genesis of colorectal carcinoma is a relatively slow process, in which the epithelium passes through a progressive series of histologically identifiable changes until it reaches a cancerous phase (Fenoglio, Pascal 1982).

The earliest histologically identifiable change is a precancerous one, with an adenomatous proliferation, resulting in the production of a benign neoplastic growth, grossly recognizable as a polyp. This is then followed by various stages of malignant transformation. In the early phases of malignant transformation, the patient can be cured of the disease before it has the chance to kill the patient. Therefore, it is important that one be able to distinguish (1) the population most at risk for developing colorectal cancer; (2) the benign non-neoplastic mucosal alterations from benign neoplastic ones; and (3) the benign neoplastic proliferations that contain potentially clinically significant cancers which may give rise to metastatic disease. Ideally, the cure of colorectal cancer depends upon the identification and removal of benign neoplastic "precancerous" tissue before it progresses to frank carcinoma (Fenoglio et al 1977).

PATIENTS AT INCREASED RISK FOR DEVELOPING COLORECTAL CARCINOMA

The persons who are at highest risk for developing colorectal carcinoma and who will do so in 100% of cases unless they undergo total proctocolectomy are patients with familial polyposis coli. These patients have a bowel which is literally carpeted with thousands of adenomatous polyps. These polyps develop in young patients and can give rise to numerous synchronous or metachronous carcinomas at an early age (Bussey 1975; DeCosse 1977; Lynch & Rush 1967; Lynch et al 1979).

Other polyposis syndromes exist beside familial polyposis coli. These include Gardner's syndrome (Gardner 1951) and Turcot's syndrome, both of which involve large numbers of adenomatous polyps and an increased incidence of colorectal carcinoma (Erbe 1976; Lynch 1979). In the latter two disorders, in addition to the intestinal polyposis, the patients manifest a variety of extra-intestinal changes. In patients with Gardner's syndrome, the extra-intestinal manifestations include epidermoid cysts, fibromas, dental abnormalities, osteomas, lymphoid polyps, abdominal desmoids, retroperitoneal fibrosis, ampullary carcinomas, and thyroid or adrenal cancers. In the case of Turcot's syndrome, the patients evidence medulloblastomas, glioblastomas, ependymomas, and carcinomas of the thyroid (Fenoglio 1984).

There are also polyposis syndromes which involve proliferations of juvenile polyps (Goodman et al 1979; Stemper et al 1975; Haggitt 1970). These patients have an increased risk of developing colorectal carcinoma, as do members of their family. However, this risk does not approach that of patients with familial polyposis, Gardner's syndrome or Turcot's syndrome.

Similarly, there is an increased risk for developing cancer in patients with Peutz-Jegher's syndrome in which hamartomatous polyps are present (Rozen, Boratz 1982).

Each of these types of polyps will be discussed subsequently (Rözen, Boratz 1982).

Other individuals who are at increased risk for developing colorectal cancer are those who have adenomatous polyps. The risk increases with increasing numbers of polyps, particularly if the patients are members of the so-called cancer syndrome families. These individuals usually have a higher than expected incidence of colorectal, endometrial, ovarian and breast cancers. Some patients with mixed adenomatous hyperplastic polyps, as defined below, also are probably at risk for the subsequent development of colorectal carcinoma.

Patients with inflammatory bowel disease are also known to be at an increased risk for developing large bowel cancer (Riddell et al 1983). This risk is stronger in patients with ulcerative colitis than in patients with regional enteritis, largely because patients with regional enteritis come to surgery sooner than those with ulcerative colitis due to the presence of numerous fistulae, perforations, and other acute abdominal catastrophes. The risk of developing carcinoma in the setting of inflammatory bowel disease will be discussed by Dr. Riddell and, therefore, is not covered in this manuscript.

Other factors that are said to be associated with an increased incidence of colorectal neoplasia involve patients who have had a ureterosigmoidostomy and then develop adenomatous and/or carcinomatous changes at the anastomotic site (Lasser, Acosta 1975; Ali 1984). It has also been suggested that there is an increased incidence of colorectal cancer in patients that have undergone previous cholecystectomy, but this is controversial (Shottenfeld, Winawer 1983; Weiss et al 1982).

NORMAL HISTOLOGY OF THE COLORECTUM

This manuscript will attempt to define the various types of polyps which may be encountered in the colon or rectum that may be associated with dysplastic or adenomatous changes and which, therefore, are presumably at increased risk for progressing to carcinoma. However, one must first understand the normal histology of the large bowel.

The wall of the colon and rectum is composed of several discrete layers that include (from the lumen outward) the mucosa, submucosa, muscularis propria, and serosa. The mucosa is composed of straight tubular glands separated by an intervening cellular lamina propria. Epithelial differentiation within the tubular glands proceeds from the base to the luminal free surface (Fenoglio et al 1977; Kaye et al 1973; Fenoglio, Pascal 1982; Fenoglio et al 1975). A mitotically active area occupies the lower one-third of the crypt and contains a population of immature cells and neuroendocrine cells (Kaye et al 1973). As the epithelial cells migrate toward the free surface, they differentiate into absorptive cells and goblet cells. Occasionally, one also encounters endocrine cells on, or near, the luminal surfaces, but they are present in vastly reduced numbers in comparison to the lower portions of the crypt.

Enveloping the crypt of Lieberkuhn is a fibroblast sheath. The fibroblasts maintain a close relationship with the epithelium and are mitotically active in the lowest one-third of the crypt, differentiating as they reach the free surface (Pascal et al 1968; Kaye et al 1968; Kaye et al 1971; Fenoglio et al 1977). The lamina propria separating the crypts of Lieberkuhn contains capillaries, plasma cells, lymphocytes, histiocytes, as well as supporting mesenchymal tissues such as fibro-blasts, collagen, and reticulin fibers.

The muscularis mucosae separates the mucosa from the submucosa. Wrapped around the muscularis mucosae is a plexus of lymphatic channels which extend as high as the bases of the crypts of Lieberkuhn, but do not extend higher into the lamina propria (Fenoglio et al 1973).

COLORECTAL POLYPS

Strictly speaking, a polyp is any bump or protrusion on the mucosal surface. This bump may be the result of a proliferation of the mucosa itself, or it may result from a proliferation of structures lying deep to the mucosa - i.e., structures in the muscularis mucosae, submucosa, muscularis propria, etc. Non-mucosal polypoid prolifer-ations give rise to lesions such as lipomas, leiomyomas, and lymphoid polyps and can be distinguished grossly, or endoscopically, from epithelial mucosal polyps.

Epithelial mucosal polyps can be divided into five major types: hyperplastic, adenomatous, mixed adenomatous-hyperplastic, hamartomatous and juvenile. These will be defined and their relationship to cancer discussed.

Hyperplastic Polyps:

Hyperplastic polyps result from an abnormality in cell division, within the crypt of Lieberkuhn, in which the replicating zone is expanded (Fenoglio et al 1977); Fenoglio, Pascal 1982; Kaye et al 1973). This results in the presence of actively dividing cells in the lower one-half of the crypt, contrasting with their restricted presence in the lower one-third of the normal mucosa. The increased mitotic activity gives rise to a larger than normal number of cells, which then results in the formation of small mucosal polyps with serrated lumens, contrasting with the straight, tubular lumens of the glands of the normal mucosa. Importantly,, although cell division is increased, there is eventual differentiation into mature adult intestinal cells (Kaye et al 1973; Fenoglio et al 1977; Fenoglio, Pascal 1982). This includes the presence of absorptive cells and goblet cells. Occasionally, the goblet cells may appear hypermature with enlarged,, engorged mucous droplets. The nuclei of the individual cells are usually round, basally placed, and show no evidence of hyperchromasia or atypia. The nuclear/cytoplasmic ratio favors the cytoplasm, particularly in the upper part of the crypt.

As in the normal mucosa, there is a partnership of the epithelium with the pericryptal fibroblast sheath (Lane et al 1971). Therefore, concomitant with the increased proliferation and hyperdifferentiation of the epithelium, there is increased proliferation and hyper-differentiation of the pericryptal fibroblasts resulting in augmented collagen production by these cells as they migrate toward the luminal surface. This results in a thickened collagen table under the free surface epithelium.

Although cellular division and mitotic activity are increased in hyperplastic polyps, it is important to recognize that division does cease in the middle of the crypt and subsequent cellular differentiation occurs. It is this restricted cellular division and subsequent cellular differentiation that distinguishes the non-neoplastic hyperplastic polyp from the neoplastic adenomatous polyp. Pure hyperplastic polyps have no apparent relationship to the subsequent development of colonic cancer.

Adenomatous Polyps (Adenomas):

As used here, the term "adenoma" encompasses a sessile, semi-sessile, or pedunculated gross growth pattern. Histologically (or grossly) the lesions may be tubular, villous, or tubulovillous (villoglandular) in configuration.

Adenomatous polyps are far less frequent than hyperplastic polyps (Fenoglio et al 1977). Like hyperplastic polyps, they arise from an abnormality in growth control with the crypt of Lieberkuhn. However, unlike the hyperplastic polyp, the abnormality is more severe, with cell division and proliferation being present throughout the entire length of the crypt, as well as on the free luminal surface. This loss of growth control leads to the production of a polyp which can range in size from several millimeters to many centimeters. Adenomatous polyps occur in all shapes and sizes and may be pedunculated, sessile or semi-sessile. However, despite their gross appearance, all are true neoplasms.

Unlike the epithelium of the normal crypt of Lieberkuhn or the epithelium lining the crypts of hyperplastic polyps, the cells lining an adenomatous crypt fail to differentiate completely into mature goblet cells and mature absorptive cells. As a result, adenomatous crypts are lined by tall cells, containing variable amounts of apical mucin, with prominent elongated or pencil-shaped hyperchromatic nuclei, arranged in a characteristic picket-fence pattern. Mitoses are usually easy to find, and atypia may be evident. Adenomatous crypts may have a tubular, papillary, or tubulovillous configuration.

The epithelial-mesenchymal partnership which exists in the normal and hyperplastic crypt of Lieberkuhn is maintained in adenomatous crypts (Kaye et al 1971; Fenoglio et al 1977). As mentioned, adenomatous epithelium is mitotically active and immature throughout the length of the crypt from the base to free surface; the same is true of the pericryptal fibroblast sheath. This results in the presence of immature fibroblasts which fail to produce their differentiated cell product, i.e., collagen, resulting in a thinning of the collagen table underlying the free mucosal surface (Lane et al 1971).

It is important to recognize that it is (1) the lack of cellular differentiation, and (2) the unrestricted cellular division that constitute the principal characteristics of neoplasia and which allow one to recognize adenomatous epithelium as being neoplastic and a precursor for the subsequent development of colorectal carcinoma.

Adenomatous Polyps with Hyperplastic Features:

There is a group of polyps which is sometimes difficult to conveniently categorize as being either hyperplastic or adenomatous (Fenoglio, Pascal 1982, Urbanski et al 1984, Fenoglio 1984). These lesions range in size, and they may be pedunculated or large sessile lesions (sometimes even villous) which characteristically have prominent intraluminal epithelial infoldings lined by large eosinophilic cells. It is the prominent "saw-toothing" of the glands which histologically creates a low-power magnification impression of a hyperplastic polyp. However, upon closer examination, many of these polyps are lined by an epithelium which is strikingly similar throughout the entire length of the intestinal crypt, suggesting that there is a failure to differentiate fully. This epithelium frequently does not resemble classic adenomatous epithelium, in that the palisaded, picket-fence arrangement may not be immediately evident. If palisading is present, the crypt lumens may be serrated rather than tubular in nature. Within these unusual polyps, these cells may contain a fair amount of cytoplasm so that the nuclear/cytoplasmic ratio may not be as high as in classic adenomas, and one has the impression of cellular eosinophilia. There may also be large amounts of mucin production in some cells.

A feature which distinguishes these proliferations from true hyperplastic polyps is that the nuclei are often not pencil-shaped but are more rounded and often are frankly dysplastic, with peripheral chromatin clumping and loss of polarity.

Another histological feature that is often useful in distinguishing between true hyperplastic polyps and adenomatous polyps with hyperplastic features appears to be the lack of the thickened collagen table under the luminal surface. As noted earlier in this discussion, there is a partnership between the crypt epithelium and the fibroblast sheath which envelops the crypt of Lieberkuhn. The fibroblastic cells of adenomatous polyps with hyperplastic features appear to be immature as evidenced by their failure to produce collagen.

Juvenile Polyps (Retention Polyps):

Juvenile polyps are generally pedunculated, non-neoplastic (perhaps hamartomatous) growths, composed of cystically dilated glands filled with mucous and inspisated inflammatory debris (Haggitt 1970). Occasionally, sessile lesions are encountered, particularly if they are small. The epithelium contains abundant mature mucin-secreting cells and absorptive cells. Neuroendocrine cells and Paneth cells may be present. Mitotic activity is usually present, particularly in the eroded areas where the epithelium may have regenerative or hyperplastic features. Individual glands are arranged in a disorderly fashion and are separated by a dense, sometimes inflamed, fibroblastic lamina propria. The inflammatory cells consist of neutrophils, eosinophils and lymphocytes. If previously eroded, stromal hemosiderin-ladened macrophages may be present.

The stalks of juvenile polyps are lined by normal mucosa and contain a submucosal core. These lesions are typically solitary, usually occurring in the rectum or sigmoid colon.

Peutz-Jegher's Polyps:

Peutz-Jegher's polyps are also pedunculated, non-neoplastic (hamartomatous) lesions that range in size from 0.1-3.0 cm in diameter and are composed of mature non-dividing intestinal epithelial cells arranged in an organized arborizing fashion around a delicate inconspicuous stroma containing bundles of smooth muscle fibers. The epithelial cells include goblet cells, absorptive cells, neuroendocrine cells and Paneth cells (Bartholomew et al 1957; Perzin et al 1983). Many fewer retention cysts are seen than in juvenile polyps, and the stroma is less conspicuous. Regenerative features may be present at the surface. Occasionally benign appearing pseudoinvasive glandular structures may be found deep in the bowel wall, in the submucosa, muscularis propria or even serosa. In some instances, continuity with the surface epithelium is evident. The benign appearance of the epithelium lining these pseudoinvasive foci distinguishes these glands from invasive carcinoma. This change has been termed "enteritis cystica profunda" (Perzin et al 1973). The stalk is lined by normal mucosa with a central submucosal core. Typically, these polyps are multiple.

RELATIONSHIP TO CANCER

Adenomatous Polyps:

There is a continuum of neoplastic changes that occur in the colon and rectum which is difficult to divide into exact subsets but which starts with the formation of a neoplastic but benign adenomatous gland (Fenoglio, Pascal 1982). The next step in the progression is the presence of cells that are cytologically malignant, yet are confined to the original contours of the crypt of Lieberkuhn without invasion of the intervening lamina propria. These areas may be classified as intraepithelial carcinoma. The next step is invasion into the lamina propria by malignant appearing glands without extension through the muscularis mucosae.

This stage might be called intramucosal carcinoma. Both intraepithelial and intramucosal carcinomas may exhibit a wide range of cellular anaplasia with both marked cytological and nuclear atypia, often accompanied by loss of cellular polarity and, occasionally, the formation of solid masses of cells within an individual gland.

A helpful diagnostic clue for the presence of areas

of severe dysplasia in this neoplastic progression is the presence of goblet cell dystrophy, in which the normally apical mucinous droplets are present in an eccentric location at the side of, or below, the atypical nuclei. It is important to note that neither intramucosal or intraepithelial carcinoma are clinically significant to the patient if all of the neoplastic tissue is removed. It is for this reason that some pathologists prefer to call polyps containing intraepithelial or intramucosal carcinoma "adenomas with severe dysplasia" or "adenomas with severe atypia."

The next step in the continuum is the presence of invasive carcinoma which is defined by the invasion through the muscularis mucosae by the malignant process. In general this invasive process is easily recognizable since the muscularis mucosae, which represents the boundary between the mucosa and submucosa, is readily identifiable, particualrly if the tissue is stained with a trichrome stain. In addition, the cellular characteristics of the lamina propria differ markedly from those in the underlying submucosa.

However, one of the most difficult diagnostic dilemmas that a pathologist can face is whether or not one is dealing with an intramucosal or an invasive cancer, particularly if the atypical cells are present in the submucosa in a lesion which has undergone erosion with pseudocarcinomatous entrapment. One reason for the difficulty in making this assessment is that, concomitant with the development of the polyp, the architecture of the muscularis mucosae may become distorted with fraying of individual muscle fibers. Thus, one may see areas of intramucosal carcinoma intermingled with these individually frayed muscle fibers, and it may be difficult to determine whether or not there is early microinvasion into the submucosa of the polyp.

In those polyps in which there is a question of the possibility of malignant invasion into the underlying submucosa, certain histological features may be helpful in making the correct diagnosis. The stromal characteristics of the normal lamina propria and submucosa are quite different, with large blood vessels usually being absent within the cellular mucosa, whereas they are abundant in the submucosa. Thus, if one sees a back-to-back glandular pattern near a large blood vessel without the surrounding characteristic lamina propria of the mucosa, one can be fairly certain that one is dealing with a truly invasive malignant process.

However, the exact diagnosis may be complicated by noninvasive areas of mucosal entrapment that undergo siderogenous desmoplasia with fibrosis and collections of hemosiderin-laden macrophages, causing the previously cellular lamina propria to appear less cellular and fibrous, more resembling submucosal tissues with a desmoplastic response to a well differentiated tumor. This dilemma can be made worse if the entrapped areas represent adenomatous glands with significant degrees of atypia.

If one has malignant cells intimately intermingled with the frayed fibers of the muscularis mucosae without clearcut evidence of submucosal invasion, the theoretic potential exists that such tumors may be capable of metastasizing when they reach this site because of the rich lymphatic plexus which invests the fibers of the muscularis mucosae and are intimately associated with it. Certainly, if one identifies a poorly differentiated carcinoma which has invaded the lymphatics in this area, serious questions need to be raised concerning the capability of such a lesion to give rise to metastases.

Carcinoma and Metastatic Disease from Colorectal Carcinomas: Prognostic Features:

The likelihood of finding an invasive carcinoma in a polyp increases with the size of the adenoma (Fenoglio et al 1977; Fenoglio, Pascal 1982). It is further influenced by the tendency of the large lesions to grow in a sessile fashion and to have villous (papillary) features. Focally, invasive carcinomas do occur in very small adenomas, either pedunculated or sessile, but this is rare. There is no known biological difference between cancers arising in villous, tubulo-villous, or tubular adenomas.

More important than the histological features are the overall gross growth pattern (sessile or pedunculated) and the depth of bowel wall penetration by the tumor (stage)

(Fenoglio, Pascal 1982). If one examines adenomatous polyps which contain areas of carcinoma and tries to relate the overall growth pattern (sessile versus pedunculated) with prognosis, one finds that the rate of metastatic disease is lower in lesions that are peduncu- lated than in those that are sessile or semi-sessile. This is an important concept since endoscopists tend to regard pedunculated and semi-sessile lesions as a single therapeutic category that can be cured by polypectomy. However, in a recent study which looked at the incidence of metastatic disease from cancers arising in adenomatous polyps with regard to gross growth pattern, it was found that the metastatic rate from sessile and semi-sessile lesions was essentially similar. In that study 3.8% of all pedunculated adenomas containing cancer had evidence of metastatic disease. This contrasted with a 30% incidence of Dukes' C lesions in semi-sessile adenomas containing cancer and a 29% incidence in sessile adenomas containing cancer (Fenoglio, Pascal 1982).

One of the reasons why the metastatic rates are similar for cancers arising in semi-sessile and sessile lesions is that a small amount of invasive carcinoma, in either growth pattern, places malignant cells in the sub- mucosa of the bowel wall, presumably giving the more deeply invasive malignant cells greater accessibility to the major lymphatic and venous drainage pathways of the colorectum. This contrasts with a similar depth of invasion in the head of a pedunculated adenoma which places the malignant cells only in the submucosa of the head of the polyp.

A second reason for the metastatic rate being so high from the semi-sessile lesions in this study is that the lesions that were looked at contained evidence of both adenomatous and carcinomatous glands. In the sessile and semi-sessile lesions, the largest proportion of tissue was composed predominantly of carcinoma with only rare residu- al adenomatous foci present, whereas in pedunculated lesions, there tended to be a greater proportion of adenomatous tissue with only a small component being carcinoma (Fenoglio, Pascal 1982). Thus, the ratio of the adenomatous to carcinomatous components within an individual polyp should be used in assessing the risk of metastatic disease. Lesions which are predominantly aden- omatous are pedunculated and contain only a small focus of carcinoma and have a lower incidence of metastatic disease than do polyps that are composed predominantly of carcinoma in which there are only a few residual adenomatous glands and are sessile or semi-sessile.

The degree of cellular differentiation is also important in assessing metastatic risk. As should be expected, the incidence of metastasis is highest in patients with poorly differentiated tumors. Of particular importance is the fact that many polyps can be predominantly composed of a well-differentiated carcinoma, but they may also contain small areas of poorly differentiated cells. Patients with polyps containing these focal, poorly differentiated areas are at an increased risk of having metastatic disease when compared with patients whose polyps are composed solely of well-differentiated carcinoma or even a moderately differentiated carcinoma. The reason for this appears to be that a poorly differentiated tumor, whether it be the predominant pattern or only a small part of the neoplasm, has a proclivity for entering lymphatics or small veins.

Finally, another feature which affects the stage of disease is the age of the patient. More than 90% of colorectal cancers occur in patients over the age of 50, but colorectal cancers are not rare in younger patients. The younger the patient, especially in the individual who is less than 40 years of age, the greater the tendency to harbor a neoplasm that may have already metastasized to the regional lymph nodes.

Mixed Adenomatous Hyperplastic Polyps and Their Relationship to Cancer:

As noted previously, mixed adenomatous hyperplastic polyps are encountered and are often difficult to diagnose. They have been reported in the literature as hyperplastic polyps (Estrada, Spjut 1980). The diagrams accompanying such papers suggest that the polyps may acquire a tubular or villous growth pattern and that there may be significant cellular dysplasia within individual crypts. If one adheres to a strict definition of the hyperplastic polyp as defined earlier and then examines the mixed adenomatous hyperplastic polyps that contain areas of severe dysplasia, carcinoma in situ or even associated foci of invasive cancers, one finds that all of the areas of dysplasia and malignant changes are present in areas not typical for the classical hyperplastic polyp (Urbanski et al 1984). Thus, it appears that it is the adenomatous or dysplastic component which may be encountered in these lesions which appear to be at risk for the subsequent development into carcinoma. How often this occurs and what the relationship is to size, location, or the age of patient has not been studied in any detail but is currently under investigation in our laboratory. My initial tendency was to discount the mixed adenomatous hyperplastic polyp as being one which might be in a potential stage of evolution to adenoma from the normal mucosa with an intermediate hyperplastic step. However, currently it is my feeling that these lesions should be viewed with caution since careful histological examination discloses that they often contain varying degrees of dysplasia, sometimes of an alarming degree, and that this dysplasia resembles that present in patients with ulcerative colitis. As in ulcerative colitis, cancers may drop off the epithelium of such lesions. Further study of this subgroup of polyps is necessary to understand their full biologic potential.

Juvenile Polyps:

Some patients have been described who have concomitant juvenile and adenomatous polyps (Smilow et al 1966; Grigioni et al 1981; Friedman, Fechner 1982). Dysplasia may also be present in individual crypts. Clearly, relatives of patients with juvenile polyps are at an increased risk for developing gastrointestinal cancers (Lynch, Rush 1967; Stemper et al 1970).

The accumulating literature suggests that juvenile polyps may undergo dysplastic changes which may then progress to frank cancer. Patients with juvenile polyps containing areas of dysplasia or adenomatous transformation should probably undergo increased surveillance to detect the malignant transformation as early as possible.

Juvenile polyps have also been described with hyperplastic features (Friedman, Fechner 1982), although the photographs in these reports suggest that "hyperplastic" areas do not have the classical features of hyperplastic

polyps but rather resemble the mixed adenomatous hyperplastic polyps described earlier.

Peutz-Jeghers Polyps:

The preneoplastic potential of Peutz-Jeghers polyps
has been debated for years with approximately 2% to 3% of
patients with the Peutz-Jeghers syndrome developing gas-
grointestinal carcinoma (Perzin, Bridge 1982). Origin
from the polyps has been suggested in some cases, although
this is not universally accepted. However, a duodenal
(Perzin, Bridge 1982) and a rectal (Miller et al 1983)
hamartomatous polyp containing areas of both adenoma and
carcinoma have been reported.

In addition, "hyperplastic" areas have been described
and illustrated in P-J polyps. The latter do not resemble
typical hyperplastic polyps but, as is the case of hyperplastic areas in juvenile polyps, more resemble the mixed
adenomatous hyperplastic polyps. Areas of dysplasia have
also been described and adequately illustrated in P-J
polyps without an intervening adenomatous change.

Part of the problem in the interpretation of the
literature on the relationship of Peutz-Jeghers polyps and
carcinomas is that many of the reports are not well illustrated, and there has been a tendency to confuse hamartomatous and adenomatous polyps (Perzin, Bridge 1982). The
presence of pseudoinvasive areas in Peutz-Jeghers polyps
further confuses the issue. Another difficulty which
arises is that patients with Peutz-Jeghers syndrome
develop their cancers in anatomic areas where the general
population develops bowel cancer most frequently (large
bowel) rather than in the commonest locations for the
hamartomas - i.e., jejuum and ileum (Miller et al 1983;
Linos et al 1981).

Hyperplastic Polyps:

To date, there is no convincing data to suggest that
hyperplastic polyps in and of themselves have any relationship to the subsequent development of cancer. This
issue, however, is confused by the recognition of polyps
with combined adenomatous and hyperplastic features, as

discussed above. Clearly the pure hyperplastic polyp is not premalignant and is quite different in histology and histogenesis from the adenomatous polyp (Fenoglio et al 1977).

In 1970 Goldman et al, introduced the concept that there were hyperplastic-like areas in 36% of adenomas smaller than 2 cm in diameter. Similar hyperplastic features were found in only 5% of lesions larger than 2 cm. This statistically important difference led them to hypothesize that hyperplastic polyps might represent a population from which some adenomas could originate. Estrada and Spjut (1980) found adenomatous areas in 13% of their hyperplastic polyps. In contrast to this, Williams et al (1980) found hyperplastic foci in only 0.6% of the adenomas examined by them, and all of the pure villous adenomas were free of hyperplastic components.

It is conceivable that the hypothesis of Hill et al (1978) may be true in some cases of the genesis of adenomatous tissue. These authors suggest that "an environmental factor A" can determine an adenomatous transformation of the colorectal mucosa in those people who are genetically predisposed to develop adenomas and that, unless this predetermining genetic factor is present, an individual is not at risk for the development of adenomatous changes. Individuals who are not genetically predisposed to develop neoplastic adenomatous tissue develop areas of hyperplasia as the result of the interaction with environmental factor A.

If this hypothesis is true, the percentage of risk for the hyperplastic epithelial changes to progress to frank cancers, or even to adenomas, has yet to be established, and thus, it remains a great problem to determine if hyperplastic epithelium demonstrates a greater dysplastic potential than the normal colonic epithelium.

Since all of the papers which describe the presence of hyperplastic colonic polyps with carcinomatous changes either describe or illustrate the presence of concomitant adenomatous or dysplastic changes, a practical approach to the problem would be as follows: (1) to assume that each of these reports presupposes that the first change is a hyperplastic one in which adenomatous or dysplastic changes may occur, and (2) the adenomatous or dysplastic changes may then themselves go on to progress to carcinoma but not the hyperplastic areas. It is important to note that no cases of carcinoma developing in pure hyperplastic polyps have yet been convincingly documented. Therefore, it would be practical to wait and do nothing further in the patient with the pure hyperplastic polyp until that patient either develops adenomatous polyps elsewhere in the colon or develops hyperplastic polyps with adenomatous or dysplastic features. If the latter should occur, then the potential for this polyp to undergo transition to carcinoma should be regarded in the same light as an adenoma or mixed adenomatous hyperplastic polyp.

CONCLUSION

There are five major types of polyps which may be encountered in the colorectum. These include hyper-plastic, adenomatous, mixed adenomatous hyperplastic, juvenile, and harmartomatous polpys. Of these, the only one which appears to have no relationship to the subse-quent develoment of carcinoma is the pure hyperplastic polyp. The adenomatous polyp has the strongest link to the subsequent development of colorectal cancer and is considered to be the precursor tissue for colorectal cancer. The predisposition to cancer is highest in patients with familial polyposis coli. The mixed adenomatous hyperplastic polyp is a little known entity that may contain significant areas of dysplasia and may be associated with areas of invasive carcinoma. These lesions need to be studied further in order to evaluate their full biologic potential. Peutz-Jeghers polyps and juvenile polyps may be associated with areas that have features resembling hyperplastic polyps, mixed adenomatous hyperplastic polyps, or adenomatous polyps. If an adeno-matous or mixed adenomatous hyperplastic polyp pattern is identified within them, they should be considered as possibly having a malignant potential analogous to the pure adenomatous polyp or the adenomatous hyperplastic polyp.

Since it is now generally accepted that adenomatous tissue represents the precursor in which carcinoma subse-quently develops in the colorectum, it follows that if this is removed one can significantly decrease the incidence of invasive cancer (Gilbertsen 1974). Indeed, the adenomacarcinoma sequence is the usual route for the development of invasive colorectal cancers, and it appears to be operational not only in the usual carcinomas of the colon but also in those instances in which carcinomas develop more frequently than in the normal population such as familial polyposis, other polyposis syndromes, or inflammatory bowel disease.

Predictive factors that may be used in estimating the likelihood of metastasis from adenomas containing cancer include growth pattern (pedunculated versus semi-sessile or sessile), patient age, cytologic differentiation, the ratio of carcinoma to adenoma within the polyp, the presence or absence of vascular involvement, and the stage of the lesion.

REFERENCES

Ali MG, Satti MG, Al-Nafussi A (1984). Multiple benign colonic polypi at the site of ureterosigmoidostomy. Cancer 53:1006.

Bartholomew LG, Dahlin DC, Waugh JM (1959). Intestinal polyposis associated with mucutaneous pigmentation (Peutz-Jeghers syndrome). Review of the literature and report of six cases with special reference to pathological findings. Gastroenterology 32:434.

Bussey HJR (1975). "Familial Polyposis Coli." Baltimore: Hopkins.

DeCosse JJ, Adams MB, Condon RE (1977). Familial polyposis. Cancer 39:267.

Erbe RW (1976). Inherited gastrointestinal polyposis syndromes. N. Eng J Med 294:1101.

Estrada RG, Spjut HJ (1980). Hyperplastic polyps of the large bowel. Am J Surg Pathol 4:127.

Fenoglio CM (submitted 1974). Diagnosing colorectal polyps. Ca-A Cancer Journal for Clinicians.

Fenoglio CM, Kaye GI, Lane N (1973). Distribution of human colonic lymphatics in normal, hyperplastic, and adenomatous tissue. Its relationship to metastasis from small carcinoms in pedunculated adenoma with two case reports. Gastroenterology 84:51.

Fenoglio CM, Kaye GI, Pascal RR, Lane N (1977). Defining the precursor tissue of ordinary large bowel carcinoma: Implications for cancer prevention. Pathol Annu 12:87.

Fenoglio CM, Pascal RR (1982). Colorectal adenomas and cancer. Pathologic relationships. Cancer 50:2601.

Fenoglio CM, Richart RM, Kaye GI (1975). Comparative electron microscopic features of normal, hyperplastic, and adenomatous human colonic epithelium II. Variations in surface architecture found by scanning electron microscopy. Gastroenterology 69:100.

Friedman CJ, Fechner RE (1982). A solitary juvenile polyp with hyperplastic and adenomatous glands. Dig Dis Sci 27:946.

Gardner EJ (1951). Genetic and clinical study of intestinal polyposisk a predisposing factor for carcinoma of the colon and rectum. Am J Hum Genet 3:167.

Gilbertsen VA (1974). Protosigmoidoscopy and polypectomy in reducing the incidence of rectal cancer. Cancer 34:936.

Goldman H, Ming S, Hickock DF (1970). Nature and significance of the hyperplastic polyps of the human colon. Arch Pathol 89:439.

Goodman ZD, Yardley JH, Milligan FD (1979). Pathogenesis of colonic polyps in multiple juvenile polyposia. Cancer 43:1906.

Grigioni WF, Alampi G, Martinelli G, Piccaluga A (1981). Atypical juvenile polyposis. Histopathology 5:361.

Haggitt RC, Pitcock JA (1970). Familial juvenile polyposis of the colon. Cancer 26:1232.

Hill MJ, Morson BC, Bussey HJR (1978). Aetiology of adenocarcinoma sequence in large bowel cancer. Lancet 1:245.

Kaye GI, Fenoglio CM, Pascal RR, Lane N (1973). Comparative electron microscopic features of normal, hyperplastic and adenomatous human colonic epithelium. Variations in cellular structure relative to the process of epithelial differentiation. Gastroenterology 64:926.

Kaye GI, Lane N, Pascal RR (1968). Colonic pericryptal fibroblast sheath: Replication, migration, and cytodifferentiation of a mesenchymal cell system in adult tissue II. Fine structural aspects of normal rabbit and human colon. Gastroenterology 54:852.

Kay GI, Lane N, Pascal RR (1971). Colonic pericrystal fibroblast sheath: Replication, migration, and cytodifferentiation of a mesenchymal cell system in adult tissue III. Replication and differentiation in the human hyperplastic and adenomatous polyps. Gastroenterology 60:515.

Lane N, Kaplan H, Pascal R (1971). Minute adenomatous and hyperplastic pllyps of the colon: Divergent patterns of epithelial growth with specific associated mesenchymal changes. Gastroenterology 60:537.

Lasser A, Acosta AE (1975). Colonic neoplasms complicating utreterosigmoidostomy. Cancer 35:1218.

Linos DA, Dozois RR, Dahlin DC, Bartholomew LG (1981). Does Peutz-Jeghers syndrome predispose to gastrointestinal malignancy? A later look. Arch Surg 116:1182.

Lynch HT, Rush AJ (1967). Heredity, polyposis, and adenocarcinoma of the colon. Gastroenterology 53:517.

Lynch HT, Lynch PM, Follett KL, Harris R (1979). Familial polyposis coli: heterogeneous polyp expression in 2 kindreds. J Med Genetics 16:1.

Miller LJ, Bartholomew LG, Dozois RR, Dahlin DC (1983). Adenocarcinoma of the rectum arising in a hamartomatous polyp in a patient with Peutz-Jeghers syndrome. Dig Dis Sci 28:1047.

Pascal RR, Kaye GI, Lane N (1968). Colonic pericryptal fibroblast sheath: Replication, migration and cytodifferentiation of mesenchymal cell system in adult tissue I. Autoradiographic studies of normal rabbit colon. Gastroenterology 54:835.

Perzin KH, Bridge MF (1982). Adenomatous and carcinomatous changes in hamartomatous polyps of the small intestine (Peutz-Jeghers syndrome): Report of a case and review of the literature. Cancer 49:971.

Perzin KH, Fenoglio CM, Pascal RR (1983). Tumors of the large and small intestine. In Silverberg D (ed): "Principles and Practice of Surgical Pathology," New York: John Wiley & Sons, Inc., pp 899.

Riddell RH, GOldman H, Ransohoff DF, Appleman HD, Fenoglio CM et al (1983). Dysplasia in inflammatory bowel disease: Standardized classification with provisional clinical implications. Human Pathol 14:931.

Rozen P, Baratz M (1982). Familial juvenile colonic polyposis with associated colon cancer. Cancer 49:1500.

Schottenfeld F, Winawer SJ (1983). Cholecystectomy and colorectal cancer. Gastroenterology 85:966.

Smilow PC, Pryor CA Jr, Swinton NW (1966). Juvenile polyposis coli. Dis Colon Rectum 9:248.

Stemper TJ, Kent TH, Summers RW (1975). Juvenile polyposis and gastrointestinal carcinoma. Ann Int Med 83:639.

Urbanski SS, Kossakowska AE, Marcon N, Bruce WR 1984). Mixed hyperplastic adenomatous polyps - an underdiagnosed entity - report of a case of adenocarcinoma arising within a mixed hyperplastic adenomatous polyp. Am J Surg Pathol 8:551.

Weiss NS, Daling JR, Ho Chow W (1982). Cholecystectomy and the incidence of cancer of the large bowel. Cancer 49:1713.

Williams GT, Arthur JF, Bussey HJR, Morson BC (1980). Metaplastic polyps and polyposis of the colorectum. Histopathology 4:155.

Carcinoma of the Large Bowel and Its Precursors, pages 45–56
© **1985 Alan R. Liss, Inc.**

HEMOQUANT - AN APPROACH TO SCREENING FOR FECAL OCCULT
BLOOD

Douglas B. McGill, M.D. and
David A. Ahlquist, M.D.
Division of Gastroenterology
Mayo Clinic
Rochester, Minnesota 55905

It is estimated by the American Cancer Society that
there will be 130,000 new cancers of the colon and rectum
in the United States in 1984. Almost half will die of
their disease in the same year and the age-adjusted U.S.
death rates per 100,000 population for 1978-1979 were 26.5
for males and 20.2 for females (Ca-A Cancer Journal for
Clinicians 1984). Modern treatment has affected the 5-
year survival very little, if at all. Ample data are
available to indicate that survival is related to the
stage when the disease is treated surgically. Since most
colorectal cancers evolve through a premalignant phase
featuring appearance and development of an adenoma or
polyp, there is the possibility that detection of these at
this early stage may favorably influence survival. Colorectal cancer therefore, fulfills the criteria of a
screenable disease (Winawer 1980). It is common, serious,
has a long presymptomatic phase, and early detection
appears to offer a favorable prognosis. An ideal screening test must be simple, convenient for patient and
screener. It must have an appropriate balance between
sensitivity and specificity. A positive test should
strongly predict the presence of disease, a negative test
predict its absence. It must, of course, be inexpensive.
Because it is likely, though not entirely certain, that
colon cancers bleed early, even as tubular adenomas,
measurement of fecal blood is potentially the most effective and cheapest screening approach.

It is important to distinguish between mass screening
of large populations and case detection or screening

individual patients for a particular disease by a personal health provider. Concerning populations, several uncontrolled screening trials have been conducted using guaiac-based tests. Firm conclusions are difficult to extract from these studies due to different experimental designs, nonstandardized assay and collection techniques, variability in diet restriction, and lack of control groups. There are ongoing randomized controlled screening trials using such tests at the University of Minnesota, Memorial-Sloan-Kettering Cancer Detection Center, University of Nottingham, and Goteburg University. Data from these studies available to date suggest that colorectal cancer is detected more frequently than in nonscreened individuals and at a more favorable pathologic stage. No study has yet demonstrated that screening reduces colon cancer-related mortality in a population. Despite these encouraging reports, one must raise serious public policy questions related to the inadequacies of the test. Thus, neither the National Cancer Institute or the American Cancer Society has recommended screening for colorectal cancer in this country with guaiac or other leuco-dye tests. In clinical practice, however, since Greegor first proposed the use of guaiac-impregnated pads in 1967, physicians have been screening or performing surveillance of their patients by performing Hemoccult determinations at the time of annual check-up examinations. Further diagnostic strategies depend on the results. Such an individual patient approach is recommended by several national groups, including the American Cancer Society (Ca-A Cancer Journal for Clinicians 1980).

Nevertheless, there remains widespread discontent with guaiac tests. Physicians use them but are deeply skeptical. Results are either positive or negative: but fecal hemoglobin is not simply present or absent. It varies continuously from amounts presumed to be "physiologic" to pathologic high levels. A fecal hemoglobin concentration above which dye tests become positive is ill-defined and there are numerous reports demonstrating insensitivity of the test to significant amounts of blood in stool (Stroehlein 1976). False-negative guaiac test results are common and lead to false reassurance. Chemical false-negatives are caused by reducing compounds such as ascorbic acid or penicillamine and, most importantly, by the conversion of heme in the gastrointestinal tract to porphyrins which do not react with the Hemoccult test.

This degradation explains the insensitivity of Hemoccult for proximal gut lesions. It also jeopardizes screening efforts based on mailed-in or stored stool specimens as heme degradation to prophyrin occurs during fecal storage. Chemical false-positive reactions are common and are due to iron, vegetable and fruit peroxidases, catalase, cytochromes, myoglobin, cimetidine, halogens, and, as indicated later, fecal water. Techniques which increase sensitivity, such as hydrating the smeared fecal aliquot, do so at the expense of their specificity. This non-specificity is magnified by multiple stool testing which frequently launches a cascade of unwarranted diagnostic procedures estimated to approach the cost of performing a barium enema on all patients screened.

In late 1983, Dr. Samuel Schwartz described the HemoQuant test which overcomes many of the technical problems with leuco-dye and cumbersome quantitative tests such as those requiring a Cr^{51} or Fe^{59} labeling (Schwartz 1983). The test is simple and straightforward, quantitative, exquisitely sensitive, specific for fecal heme, and suitable for automation. It also recognizes the intestinal degradation of heme which, as pointed out by Schwartz, was anticipated in 1921 by Snapper and co-workers who emphasized the finding of negative guaiac reactions in the feces of patients known to have gross intestinal bleeding. Subsequently such feces were found to exhibit intense red fluorescence on appropriate light exposure and fecal extracts had absorption bands characteristic of porphyrins or altered hemes or both. The chemical basis of the HemoQuant test is the chemical conversion of iron-containing nonfluorescing heme to fluorescent porphyrins lacking iron. Following solvent extraction the porphyrins are measured in a fluorescent spectrophotometer and the results expressed as milligram of hemoglobin equivalents per gram of feces. That is, the values are directly equal to the amount of hemoglobin required to yield the amounts of porphyrin found rather than to the actual amount of hemoglobin present as such in the fecal sample. Assuming a serum hemoglobin concentration of 15 g/dL and a fecal output per day of 150 grams, 1 mg/g of feces is roughly equivalent to blood loss of 1 mL of blood/24 hours. The assay uses an 8 mg sample of feces which is heated in oxalic acid:Fe SO4, thereby converting fecal heme to porphyrins and retaining those porphyrins that were formed from heme in the intestinal tract - or during storage.

The solvent extraction sequence recovers over 95% of the heme-derived porphyrins and removes more than 99% of contaminating compounds, including coproporphyrin and chlorophyll. This fraction, therefore, assays the total equivalent concentration of hemoglobin. A second aliquot is heated in a citric acid reagent which solubilizes and assays only those prophyrins that were formed from heme in the intestinal tract. This intestinal converted fraction can be expressed as a percentage of the total. The test has been extensively validated chemically. Figure 1 shows the correlation of HemoQuant results, that is, the total or oxalic acid fraction against measurements by high performance liquid chromatography.

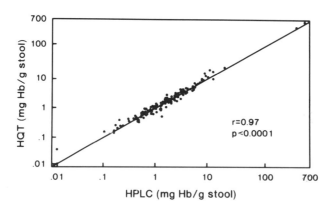

Fig. 1. Correlation of "Hb equivalent" values by chromatography and HemoQuant. Schwartz S, et al. Clin Chem 29:2064, 1983.

Recovery of hemoglobin added to feces averages 99.1% of theoretical values. Reproducibility is excellent. In a later report Schwartz and Ellefson reported on HemoQuant values in nine normal volunteers who drank 10-36 mL of their own blood (Schwartz 1984). Recovery was 88% by HemoQuant but Hemoccult tests remained negative despite the more than twenty-fold increase in fecal heme. Up to 83% of the ingested heme was converted in the intestinal tract as recognized in the citric acid fraction. Approximately 25% of the heme in ingested meat was recovered in feces, whereas negligible amounts of heme were found in fish and fowl while their ingestion led to no significant increase in fecal heme. Control fecal values represented an average of approximately 0.5 mL of blood per day.

In collaboration with Schwartz and others, we undertook further validation of the HemoQuant test and compared it directly with Hemoccult in over 1000 consecutive stool specimens which had been sent to a clinical laboratory for occult blood determination (Ahlquist 1984). Quantities of blood ranging from 0.1-14 mg of hemoglobin/g of stool were added to 27 randomly selected stools. Recovery was not affected by the addition of high concentrations of ferrous sulfate (24 mg/g stool) or of cimetidine (10 mg/g stool). Each compound was added to separate aliquots of five stools with low hemoglobin concentrations, that is, < 2 mg/g. All stools containing these additives became Hemoccult- positive. HemoQuant recovery was not altered by ascorbic acid added to stools with more than 7 mg hemoglobin/g, yet Hemoccult reactions were inhibited in all. The intestinal converted fraction was proportional to HemoQuant values, further confirmation that this fraction is a metabolic product of heme. (Fig. 2).

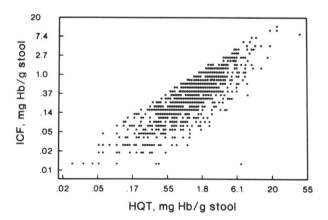

Fig. 2. HemoQuant results in 1018 patient stool specimens. HQT refers to total mg of Hb/stool, ICF to that portion converted to porphyrin during intestinal transit. Ahlquist DA, et al. Ann Int Med 101:298,, 1984.

A number of conditions were evaluated with respect to their effect on both Hemoccult and HemoQuant results. These included, in addition to those already mentioned, the effects of stool consistency, aqueous dilution, and storage. A subjective grading system of stool liquidity was developed and validated against measurements of dry weight. Hemoccult reactivity was found to depend directly on water content of stools. Thirty-three percent of tests were positive with liquid stools (n=15), but fell progressively with increasing dryness to 14.8% with semi-liquid (n=88), 7.9% with soft (n=140), 3.9% with formed (n=710), and only 1.5% with hard (n=65) stools. At any fecal hemoglobin concentration wetter stools were more apt to be Hemoccult-positive than were drier stools. (Fig.3).

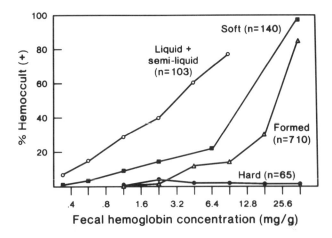

Fig. 3. Factors influencing Hemoccult reactivity: Native hydration. Ahlquist DA, et al. Ann Int Med 101:299,1984.

Hemoccult reactivity was altered significantly by homogenization of stools with increasing amounts of water. Hemoccult-negative tests almost always became positive after serial aqueous dilution. This occurred despite hemoglobin concentrations as low as 0.2 mg/g or less. These dilutional concentrations were precisely recognized by HemoQuant. Hydration of the stool once smeared on the Hemoccult pad had much less effect. When tested on freshly smeared stools pad hydration did not alter the results.

From 502 consecutive fresh stools tested with both the hy-
drated and nonhydrated techniques, Hemoccult was positive
in 48 with both, in 10 with hydration only, and in 7 with
nonhydration only.   In a separate experiment similar hydration did augment Hemoccult reactivity of stools stored
on the pads for 24 hours, as has been recognized by
others.   Of 18 initially Hemoccult-positive stools only 12
were still positive without hydration, while 17 were
positive with hydration.   The effect of storage time and
temperature was assessed on specimens analyzed after
periods of up to 16 days of storage at -20 C.; 4, 25 and
38 degrees C.   HemoQuant values representing the sum of
degraded heme plus residual heme were not influenced by
storage time or temperature. (Fig. 4A).   However, heme
degradation progressed during storage at 4 degrees or
higher as the converted fraction accounted for an
increasing percentage of total heme equivalents (Fig. 4B)
and, therefore, Hemoccult positivity decreased. (Fig 4C).

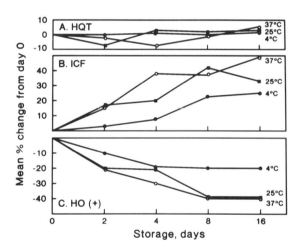

Fig. 4.   Effect of storage time and temperature on:
Fig. 4A - HemoQuant.
Fig. 4B - Converted fraction (ICF).
Fig. 4C - Hemoccult.
Ahlquist DA, et al.   Ann Int Med 101:300, 1984.

The intestinal converted fraction accounted for significantly more fecal hemoglobin in 132 Hemoccult-negative stools than in 27 Hemoccult-positive stools with means of 38% and 19%, respectively, (p<.0001). The HemoQuant concentrations in these experiments were from 3.2 to 25.6 mg/g. For all stools, as shown in Figure 5, as the proportion of degraded fecal heme increases Hemoccult positivity decreased.

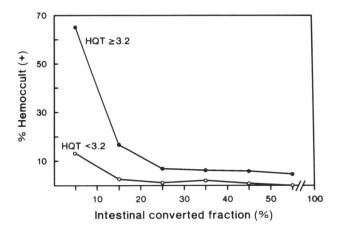

Fig. 5. Effect of heme degradation on Hemoccult positivity. Ahlquist DA, et al. Ann Int Med 101:299, 1984.

The intestinal converted fraction over-all contributed importantly to HemoQuant measurements and the median fraction was 32% with the range of 1-98%. The sensitivity of Hemoccult at different HemoQuant levels was examined. (Fig. 6).

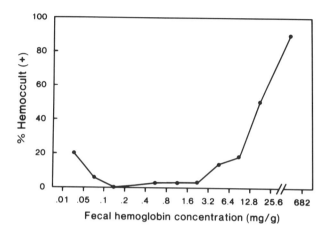

Fig. 6. Effect of Fecal Hb concentration on Hemoccult positivity. Ahlquist DA, et al. Ann Int Med 101:299, 1984.

Hemoccult was positive in only 17.9% of stools showing HemoQuant values between 6.4 and 12.8 mg and in 50% of stools between 12.8 and 25.6 mg/g stool. The highest fecal hemoglobin level undetected by Hemoccult was 42.5 mg/g. Yet Hemoccult yielded a positive reaction with concentrations as low as 0.04 mg hemoglobin/g stool.

We concluded that HemoQuant reliably quantifies fecal heme and is unaffected by substances which interfere with guaiac tests. The intestinal converted fraction is not detected by Hemoccult and frequently constitutes the major portion of fecal heme. Hemoccult reactivity is strongly dependent on fecal water content, while fecal storage causes a progressive loss of Hemoccult reactivity due to heme degradation, but does not alter HemoQuant results. The normal variations of fecal liquidity and heme degradation likely explain most chemical hemoccult false-positive and false-negative reactions.

How will HemoQuant be used clinically? Several questions remain. With a quantitative test one must begin with definition of normal. It is extremely difficult to identify a normal concentration of fecal hemoglobin. Ethical, as well as logistic and financial considerations, argue against complete examinations of the gastrointestinal tract in presumably healthy volunteers. Therefore, without such studies (or even with them) a bleeding lesion such as a colon polyp, gastric erosion, or arteriovenous malformation, can never be excluded with certainty in a person thought to be healthy. Radio-chromium studies have suggested that up to 2 mL of blood/24 hours may be lost through the gastrointestinal tract. The Mayo Clinic group reported that in a group of presumed healthy controls median HemoQuant was 1.19. In those not taking aspirin the median value was 0.68, and if the subjects were not eating red meat and not taking aspirin the median value was 0.22 mg/g stool (Ahlquist 1984). Four percent of these controls were Hemoccult-positive. Vigorous physical activity, such as jogging, may produce increased "normal" fecal blood loss. As recently shown, fecal hemoglobin levels as measured by HemoQuant increased in 20 of 24 runners after a marathon (Stewart 1984). The mean fecal hemoglobin concentration was 1.08 mg/g (range 0.11-2.36) in controls, 0.9 mg/g (0.18-2.41) in runners before a race, but peaked at 3.96 mg/g (0.37-43.2) after a race. (Fig. 7).

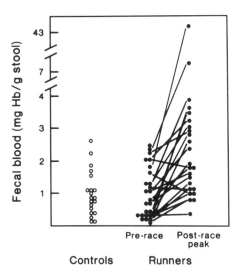

Fig. 7. Fecal blood levels of conditioned runners before and after a long distance race, and of nonrunning controls. Stewart et al. Ann Int Med 100:844, 1984.

HemoQuant has been applied to patients with bleeding or potentially bleeding gastrointestinal lesions (Ahlquist 1984). Blood loss was $\geq$ 2 mg/g in 76% of patients with polyps $\geq$ 2 cm (n=12), and in 93% of all colon cancers (n=30). The intestinal converted fraction tended to be higher as expected in patients with proximal lesions compared to those with lesions low in the colon. Thus, HemoQuant can discriminate controls from patients with gastrointestinal malignancies and other hemorrhagic lesions and screening HemoQuant values >2 likely reflect gastrointestinal pathology. Many more patients need to be studied in order to further define critical values. Obviously, the higher the value the more likely there is disease.

Fecal blood tests all share certain drawbacks with respect to screening for colorectal cancer. They are not esthetic. Positivity may be related to lesions other than colorectal cancer. Bleeding patterns of colorectal cancers are not yet known, but cancers may not bleed continuously or excessively, particularly when small. Less is known about the bleeding patterns of polyps. Even when detected at the stage of occult bleeding the lesions may be relatively far advanced. Ideally the diagnosis would be made earlier. On the other hand, other indirect tests such as those on serum using monoclonal antibodies directed against tumors are not yet sufficiently well developed, while more direct diagnostic tests such as barium enema and colonoscopy are too cumbersome for screening. Periodic surveillance with these procedures under certain circumstances is appropriate, while efforts continue to identify an inexpensive and effective screening test suitable for all individuals and populations. HemoQuant appears superior to guaiac-based and immunochemical tests. Several additional studies are being done to validate its usefulness. Automation is under development. We are evaluating sampling techniques. Prior to widespread clinical use further studies will have to determine an appropriate threshold level of sensitivity below which individuals can be presumed to be normal and above which further investigation is required.

REFERENCES

Ahlquist DA, McGill DB, Owen RA, Young DS, Taylor WF, Beart RS Jr, Center CL, Schwartz S (1983). A new quantitative assay for fecal hemoglobin, Hemoquant. Analyses in Health and GI Disease. (Abstract) GE 84:1089.

Ahlquist DA, McGill DB, Schwartz S, Taylor WF, Ellefson M, Owen RA (1984). HemoQuant, a new quantitative assay for fecal hemoglobin: Comparison with Hemoccult. Ann Int Med 101:297.

American Cancer Society. "Guidelines for the cancer-related checkup. Recommendations and rationale" (Jul/Aug 1980). Ca-A A Cancer Journal for Clinicians. 30(4).

American Cancer Society. "Cancer Statistics, 1984" (Jan/FEb 1984). Ca-A Cancer Journal for Clinicians. 34(1).

Schwartz S, Dahl J, Ellefson M, Ahlquist DA (1983). The "HemoQuant" Test: A specific and quantitative determination of heme (hemoglobin) in feces and other materials. Clin Chem 29:2061.

Schwartz S, Ellefson M (1983). Fecal recovery of hemo-proteins from blood, meat, and fish ingested by normal volunteers: The HemoQuant assay. (Abstract). GE 84:1032.

Stewart JG, Ahlquist DA, McGill DB, Ilstrup DM, Schwartz S, Owen RA (1984). Gastrointestinal blood loss and anemia in runners. Ann Int Med 100:843.

Stroehlein JR, Fairbanks VF, McGill DB, GO VLW (1976). Hemoccult detection of fecal occult blood quantitated by radioassay. Am J Dig Dis 21:841.

Winawer SJ, Schottenfeld D, Sherlock P (1980). "Colo-rectal cancer: Prevention, epidemiology, and screening." Vol. 13, Progress in Cancer Research and Therapy.

Carcinoma of the Large Bowel and Its Precursors, pages 57–63
© **1985 Alan R. Liss, Inc.**

VEGETABLE PEROXIDASE INHIBITOR - AN IMPROVEMENT IN THE
GUAIAC FECAL OCCULT BLOOD TEST

Martin Fleisher, Ph.D., Carol Smith, B.S.,
Sidney J. Winawer, M.D.*, and Morton K.
   Schwartz, Ph.D.
Department of Clinical Chemistry
*Gastroenterology Service, Dept. of Medicine
Memorial Sloan-Kettering Cancer Center
New York, NY 10021

Colorectal cancer is one of the highest incident
cancers in the U.S., accounting for more than 130,000 new
cases each year. This fact, along with the high mortality
rate, has stimulated interest in new screening tests and
diagnostic procedures for the early detection of the
disease.

The fecal occult blood test (FOBT), based on guaiac
oxidation, is a widely used screening test for blood in
stool. The application of the FOBT in a prescribed way
was popularized by Greegor (Greegor 1967) who recommended
the use of six slides over a 3-day period, testing two
slides per stool specimen on a meat-free, high bulk diet.
In his initial studies, colorectal cancer was detected in
patients at an early pathological stage. Since a positive
test for occult blood in stool is possibly due to colorectal cancer or premalignant polyps, special attention
must be paid to test conditions. In particular, those
conditions which affect test specificity, resulting in an
increase in false-positive reaction, need to be identified
and eliminated. The conditions and recommendations for
FOB testing have recently been reviewed (Gnauck, Macrae,
Fleisher 1984).

A positive guaiac occult blood test is caused by the
phenolic oxidation of the guaiac to a blue compound,
facilitated by the peroxidase-like action of hemoglobin
(Figure 1).

Peroxidase-like activity of $H_g b$

$$Hb + 2H_2O_2 \longrightarrow 2H_2O + O_2$$

Oxidation of Guaiac

$$O_2 + guaiac \longrightarrow Oxidized \ guaiac$$

(colorless)   (blue)

Figure 1. Principle of phenolic oxidation of guaiac in the presence of hemoglobin (Hb).

Rehydration of slides leads to an apparent improvement in test sensitivity, presumably due to a more intimate contact between hemoglobin and guaiac and/or an enhanced pseudoperoxidase activity of hemoglobin. (Fleisher, Schwartz, Winawer 1980). False positivity ranges from 2% for unhydrated slides to 20% for slides rehydrated prior to development (Winawer 1982).

However, rehydration may also affect the specificity of the FOBT by increasing false-positive results produced by food POD in the stool. Individual foods such as turnip (Baumel et al 1979), pineapple (Baumel et al 1979), banana (Adlercreutz 1978), and uncooked vegetables (Bassett 1980) are stated to be especially likely to produce false-positive results. The effect of peroxidase levels in food and its relative impact on colorectal cancer screening have been studied (Caligiore 1982). Foods were grouped according to peroxidase activity equivalent to 1.0 mg of blood. Table 1 lists some foods containing the greatest peroxidase activity. It is estimated that false positivity due to dietary interferences ranges between 0.5 to 2%.

Table 1

Food with Peroxidase (POD) Activity Equivalent to 1.0 ml of Blood (Caligiore 1982).

Amount of Food with POD Activity Equivalent to 1.0 ml Blood (g)	Food Items
5	Broccoli, Turnip
5-10	Cauliflower, Red Radish, Parsnip, Cantaloups
10-20	Cucumber, Mushroom, Parsley, Zucchini
20-50	Cabbage, Potato, Carrot, Grapefruit

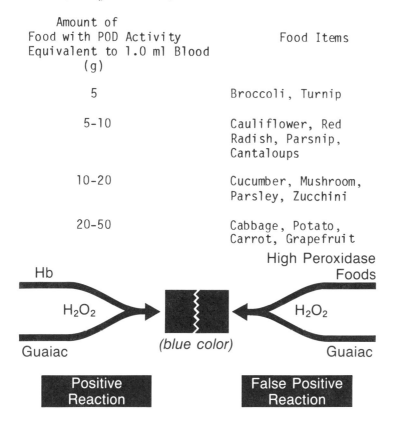

Figure 2. Principle of pholic oxidation of guaiac in the presence of Hb and food peroxidases treated with H₂O₂. Note false-positive reaction resulting from food peroxidase reaction.

A recently introduced modification of the guaiac impregnated paper FOBT may eliminate the need for special dietary restrictions for proper test performance. This new test, referred to as ColoScreen VPI (Helena Laboratories, Beaumont, Texas), selectively inhibits vegetable and fruit peroxidase interferences. Figures 2 and 3 demonstrate the principle of vegetable peroxidase interference and the inhibitory effect of the vegetable peroxidase blocking reagent.

The addition of the vegetable peroxidase inhibitor (VPI) to a ColoScreen slide containing a stool specimen in which vegetable or fruit POD are absent does not affect the reactivity of hemoglobin if present (Figure 2). In the event vegetable or fruits POD are present in the stool, the addition of VPI selectively inhibits the reaction due to POD.

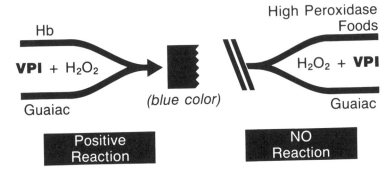

Figure 3. Effects of ColoScreen VPI on dietary interference. The reaction of Hb in the presence of
guaiac, H_2O_2 and VPI results in a true positive
reaction. However, the food peroxidase
interference is blocked by VPI preventing
reaction of guaiac and H_2O_2 which would
otherwise yield a false-positive test.

This unique concept utilizing a specific blocking reagent for interfering compounds may lead to an increase in specificity and sensitivity of the FOBT. Laboratory tests on ColoScreen VPI using stool specimens spiked with human hemoglobin (HHB) and horseradish peroxidase (HPOD) have indicated the effectiveness of this reagent in blocking POD interference (Table 2). Spiked stool specimens were applied to the ColoScreen VPI slide in the usual manner and were permitted to dry. This simulates the actual collection procedure followed by the patient. Two drops of vegetable peroxidase inhibitor (VPI) were applied to each specimen window followed by the addition of H_2O_2 developer.

Specimens containing HHb alone produced a moderately positive color response (graded in our laboratory as a +3). Peroxidase (HPOD)-containing specimens treated with VPI produced no color response. Specimens containing HPOD but NOT treated with VPI prior to the addition of developer produced a moderately positive reaction. A mixture of HHb and HPOD gave a positive reaction indicating the selective inhibition of HPOD by the VPI without affecting the HHb present in the stool specimen. Hence, the selective inhibition of food peroxidases can be accomplished by treating the ColoScreen Slide with VPI prior to development.

TABLE 2

EFFECT OF VEGETABLE PEROXIDASE INHIBITOR (COLOSCREEN VPI) ON FOBT

SPECIMEN COMPOSITION

	STOOL + HHb	STOOL + HPOD	STOOL + Hb + HPOD
DEVELOPING REAGENT ONLY	MODERATELY POSITIVE	MODERATELY POSITIVE	MODERATELY POSITIVE
COLOSCREEN VPI REAGENT FOLLOWED BY DEVELOPING REAGENT	MODERATELY POSITIVE	NEGATIVE	MODERATELY POSITIVE

The elimination of vegetable peroxidase interference is a major step in improving FOBT specificity. A lower false-positive rate would reduce the risk and costs associated with the diagnostic follow-up of positive FOBT. The relationship of false-positive FOBT to life expectancy and associated increases in diagnostically related cost are shown in Table 3. These conclusions are based on computer models utilizing presently available data and other reasonable assumptions.

TABLE 3

EFFECT OF HEMOCCULT FALSE POSITIVE RATE: COST-
EFFECTIVENESS MEASURES, 50-YEAR OLD, AVERAGE RISK WOMAN
(EDDY, 1980)

False-Positive Rate (%)	Life Expectancy (days)	Increased Cost of Differential Diagnosis (dollars)
1	74.54	66.81
5	74.41	330.11
10	74.25	659.23

The importance in decreasing or eliminating false-positivity in FOBT vis a vis cost effectiveness is suggested from this data.

The "simple" slide test for fecal occult blood as a possible screening tool for colorectal cancer is, in reality, exceedingly complex. The two major controversial aspects of the FOBT, effects of diet and rehydration on test specificity can be effectively addressed and tested. Since opinions remain divided as to the desirability of rehydrating slides (without imposing strict dietary controls) in screening programs (Gilbertsen 1980; Winawer 1980), the use of ColoScreen VPI would eliminate the main concerns and difficulties of imposing dietary restrictions as a screening criteria.

It is apparent from the considerations presented above that if the FOBT is to be used successfully improvements in both sensitivity and specificity leading to an improvement in the predictive value is essential and welcomed.

REFERENCES

Adlercreutz H, Liewendehl K, Virkola P (1978). Evaluation of Fecatest, a new guaiac test for occult blood in feces. Clin Chem 24:756-761.

Bassett ML, Goulston KJ (1980). False positive and negative Hemoccult reactions on a normal diet and effect of diet restrictions. Aust NZ J Med 10:1-4.

Baumel H, Giraudon M, Deizonne B, Rey MH (1979). Depistage des tumeurs colo-rectales: Interet du test clinique au guaiac. Med Chir Dig 8:307-312.

Caligiore P, Macrae FA, St. John DJB, Rayner LJ, Legge JW (1982). Peroxidase levels in food: relevance to colorectal cancer screening. Amer J Clin Nutrition 35:1487-1489.

Eddy DM (1980). Computer models and the evaluation of colon cancer screening programs, in Winawer SJ, Schottenfeld D, Sherlock P (eds). Colorectal Cancer· Prevention, epidemiology, and screening. New York, Raven Press pp 285-298.

Fleisher M, Schwartz MK, Winawer SJ (1980). Laboratory studies on the Hemoccult slide for fecal occult blood testing in colorectal cancer, In Winawer SJ, Schottenfeld D, Sherlock P (eds) Colorectal cancer: Prevention, epidemiology, and screening. New York, Raven Press, pp 181-187.

Gilbertsen VA, Church TR, Grewe FJ et al (1980). The design of a study to assess occult blood screening for colon cancer. J Chronic Dis, 33:107-114.

Gnauck R, Macrae FA, Fleisher M (1984). How to perform the fecal occult blood test. Ca-A Cancer Journal for Clinicians. 34:134-147.

Greegor DH (1967). Diagnosis of large bowel cancer in the asymptomatic patient. JAMA 201:943-945.

Winawer SJ, Fleisher M, Baldwin M, Sherlock P (1982). Current status of fecal occult blood testing in screening for colorectal cancer. 32:3-15.

Winawer SJ, Andrews M, Flehinger B et al (1980). Progress report on controlled trial of fecal occult blood testing for the detection of colorectal neoplasia. Cancer 45: 2959-2964.

Carcinoma of the Large Bowel and Its Precursors, pages 65–76
© 1985 Alan R. Liss, Inc.

SCREENING FOR COLORECTAL CANCER: THE RATIONALE AND A
RECENT ADVANCE IN THE DETECTION OF FECAL OCCULT BLOOD

William G. Friend, M.D.
Clinical Assistant Professor of Surgery
University of Washington
Seattle, Washington 98104

HISTORICAL REVIEW AND RATIONALE

Cancer of the colon and rectum may be the most important malignant disease in this country. As a cause of death, it is second only to lung cancer in men. It is the third leading lethal malignancy in women. About a half-million of our current population have been diagnosed as having colorectal cancer, and almost 60,000 deaths per year are attributed to this type of cancer (Cancer Facts and Figures 1984; Levin 1974).

An estimated 130,000 new cases are identified annually and a substantial majority of these patients are presenting with symptoms, a condition which correlates all too well with poor prognosis for cure and survival. Over half of all cases presenting with symptoms are also presenting with metastases and/or regional lymph node involvement, circumstances which are associated with a five-year survival rate of less than 50% (Murphy 1977; Silverberg 1984). In contrast, 95% of asymptomatic patients have tumors which are still localized and, in these cases, the survival rate is of the order of 90% in some series of patients (Hertz et al 1960; Axtell 1976; Murphy 1977). The value of being able to detect these malignancies while patients are still asymptomatic is evident.

Early detection and diagnosis of colorectal cancer throughout a large population thus represents a major opportunity. It has been estimated that treatment of tumors in asymptomatic patients could save 40,000 lives per year (Winawer 1984). However, despite the recognition of this opportunity for many years, the problem of achieving widespread screening has been persistently resistant to resolution. Since Dukes' classic report in 1932, which strongly suggested the potential benefit of detecting the presence of rectal cancers while they are still confined to the intestinal wall, there has been neither an appreciable increase in the proportion of localized tumors detected nor an appreciable improvement in mortality rates (Table 1). Among Dukes' patients, 18% of the tumors were classified as stage A and 35% as B (Dukes 1932). Among the patients surveyed in a nationwide audit by the Commission on Cancer of the American College of Surgeons, the incidence of localized tumors was between 28.2% and 30.5%, while all the rest had either invaded the pericolic fat, involved regional lymph nodes, or had distant metastases, Table 2 (Murphy 1977). Current 5-year survival rates for localized tumors range from 73% to 88% as compared to 25% for tumors that have spread beyond the wall of the intestine (Cancer Facts and Figures 1984; Murphy 1977). Thus, since less than half of all colorectal cancers are localized at first diagnosis, and since survival rates have improved only slightly despite the introduction of combination chemo-, radiation and immunotherapy as well as improved surgical techniques, the development of a means of early detection appears to have the most promise of reducing mortality due to colorectal cancer.

TABLE 1

Dukes - 1932

	Incidence	Survival Rate*
A	18%	90%
B	35%	80%
C	47%	25%

* 3 year survival rate.

TABLE 2

Murphy - 1977

28.2% - 30.5% -- Localized
20.6% - 22.3% -- Invasion of pericolic fat
 9.5% - 12.0% -- Spread to regional lymph nodes
14.0% - 16.0% -- Invasion of pericolic tissues and nodes
20.3% - 25.5% -- Distant metastases

Three methods of screening for early detection - rectal digital palpation, sigmoidoscopy and testing for occult fecal blood - have been available for years and, in some instances, centuries. All three procedures have their benefits and deficiencies, but the one most recently developed, the detection of occult fecal blood, may be adequate as a broad screening tool.

Digital rectal examination is increasingly done as a routine element of conventional physical examinations and it is estimated that about one-third of all persons over 45 years receive rectal examinations each year. The utility and limitation of this procedure is that, although it can detect many cancers of the rectum, these cancers represent only 16%-20% of colorectal cancers. Further, it may miss some rectal cancers because of their small size or because they are obscured by stool or feces.

Sigmoidoscopy with the rigid 25 cm instrument can explore considerably more of the colon, and has been utilized since before the turn of the century. Walsh and Spiro (1981), from a review of the literature, note that sigmoidoscopy successfully identifies 90% of tumors present in the rectum and rectosigmoid colon (a false negative rate of 10%), but only 40% of tumors in the sigmoid colon (a false negative rate of 60%). They also observed that, in their series of symptomatic patients with histologically confirmed carcinoma at the recto-sigmoid junction, the rate of detection by the combined use of digital and sigmoidoscopic examination was only 46.2%. Adding radiologic examination with a barium enema to the two screening procedures increased the number of positive identifications to 76.9%. For reason of its in-ability to detect proximal colorectal cancers, and due to the fact that it is relatively expensive, uncomfortable, and bears some small risk of bowel perforation, sigmoidoscopy has never been suitable for wide-scale screening.

The third method of screening, testing for occult fecal blood, has many distinct advantages and the potential capability of great screening utility. It has the inherent capacity to detect tumors present at any position in the entire length of the colon. It is noninvasive, safe, inexpensive and does not produce any discomfort. Most importantly, since gross blood in the stool is the chief complaint of patients who have cancer of the colon and rectum, the detection of occult fecal blood at an earlier stage could theoretically identify 90% of patients with these tumors. Nonetheless, despite the existence for over 20 years of methods for detecting occult fecal blood, most people with colorectal cancer have never been screened for occult blood in their stools nor have they had a rectal examination. The vast majority of patients with colorectal cancer still come to their physicians because of visible fecal blood.

Obviously, the conventional and most frequently used test for occult fecal blood, which depends on the reaction between blood and guaiac, has not been used frequently enough to shift a significant proportion of identified tumors from Dukes' C stage toward Dukes' a stage. A variety of reasons have contributed to our failure to have made optimum use of this method for screening large numbers of asymptomatic people. Some of these relate to the criteria for determining whether a disorder is worthy of mass screening. Other reasons relate to characteristics of the target population and the capabilities of the screening procedure itself.

The criteria for the suitability of a disorder for screening have been outlined (Cole and Morrison 1980), and colorectal cancer meets all of them. The first criteria are that the disorder be reasonably common within a population and that it have serious consequences. As we have seen, very substantial absolute numbers of people will develop these malignancies and die because of them. However, because of a relatively low prevalence of 3 per 1,000 asymptomatic people over 55 (Kristein 1980), neither of these facts may be as widely recognized by the target population as may be required. There may be insufficient awareness of colorectal cancer and thus, not enough motivation for large-scale use and compliance with a screening procedure. Colorectal cancer also meets the criteria of having an asymptomatic phase during which screening methods are capable of detecting it, and the availability of treatment which, if used during this phase, is capable of favorably influencing patient survival and/or function. Lastly, adequate health services are available to provide follow-up of the projected number of positive screening tests. The capacity to diagnostically confirm positive tests and effectively treat patients with confirmed colorectal cancer is currently present.

One of the major problems of developing an effective screening program relates to differences between patients who seek medical aid for complaints, and people who are apparently well but who may benefit from the early discovery of an as yet asymptomatic condition. Patients expect, and should receive, the full leverage of diagnostic procedures required to help make them well again. In contrast, apparently healthy people do not feel compelled to be excessively inconvenienced, discomforted, subjected to risk, or be charged for procedures which may protect them from illness which only might befall them. Thus, a screening procedure, to be acceptable to large numbers of people, must incur minimal inconvenience, discomfort, risk and cost (Diehl 1981).

The second main set of criteria concern the accuracy of the methodology. The test must have adequate sensitivity, specificity and efficiency if it is to have good predictability. Excessive incidence of false positive results incur unnecessary cost, inconvenience, and alarm for the individual patient. Excessive false negatives obviously diminish the effectiveness of screening.

Most of the tests for occult blood are based on the use of guaiac, although some have utilized benzidine or orthotolidine. The chemical reaction involved is not completely understood, but is basically no different in today's methods than it was in the original tests developed over one hundred years ago. Hemoglobin has activity which, like peroxidase, reacts with hydrogen peroxide with the production of free oxygen radicals.

These, in turn, react with guaiac to form blue-colored quinone-like substances, thus indicating a positive test.

The first chemical test to be used by the medical profession to detect occult blood was known as the bench guaiac test, and it was cumbersome. Powdered guaiac was first freshly dissolved in alcohol, mixed with glacial acetic acid and hydrogen peroxide, and this mixture applied to a fecal sample. Small wooden sticks were used to take samples from stools. Physicians in hospitals took samples this way. Outpatients also used sticks to take samples, and then saved the specimens in their refrigerator until they could be brought to the doctor's office or hospital laboratory. Even the most widely used tests today require the use of the little stick although the rest of the procedure has been much improved upon.

The first modification in the bench guaiac test was the elimination of the use of acetic acid, when it was realized that it was not necessary. This allowed a solution of guaiac in alcohol to be loaded onto a square of filter paper and allowed to dry. This gave rise to the first commercial slide test, Hemoccult. To use this test, the stool sample was applied to the guaiac-impregnated filter paper with a wooden applicator. These slides were then sent to the physician, where the developer solution of hydrogen peroxide and alcohol was applied and the test was read. Subsequently, test kits which included the developing solution were introduced commercially. These allowed patients to do the entire test at home.

This last improvement provided several benefits. It obviated the need for storage of samples in the refrigerator, and it obviated the need for rehydrating the samples in the laboratory or physician's office. This last is particularly meaningful since the rehydration was done because the test was thought to be less sensitive on dried fecal samples. Subsequently, it was determined that rehydration increased the test sensitivity unduly and led to excessive false positives.

Postive guaiac tests can indicate bleeding from sources other than colorectal cancer such as duodenal or gastric ulcers, hemorrhoids, ulcerative colitis and any of a variety of other bleeding lesions of the gastrointestinal tract. Additionally, it is thought by many that the hemoglobin in red meat and peroxidase in some vegetables and fruits can lead to false positives. From the available evidence, it is not clear that dietary control is as meaningful today as was once believed.

The detection of fecal occult blood by presently available methods requires an estimated daily loss of blood of 10 to 20 ml, which will result in levels of greater than 2 ml of blood per 100 gm of stool (Stroehlein et al 1978) or 1.5 - 3 mg of hemoglobin per gram of stool (Barrows et al 1978). Estimates of false positives with Hemoccult tests range from 8% (Stroehlein et al 1978) to less than 2%, even in patients who observe no dietary restrictions (Ostrow et al 1973). It has also been observed that ingestion of aspirin may produce false positives by encouraging bleeding from the intestinal wall. Cimetidine has also been observed to produce false negatives, although the mechanism by which it does so is not known.

Occult blood tests are not intended for people with gross rectal bleeding, whether from bleeding cancers or bleeding hemorrhoids. If a person can already see red blood on the stool or on the toilet tissue for any reason, he or she is not a candidate for any type of occult blood test.

False negatives are also a concern in any screening procedure, and they are very difficult to estimate since negative test results in asymptomatic patients are rarely followed up with further diagnostic procedures. Occult blood testing does have a small percentage of false negatives (Songster et al 1980), and this may be due to a number of factors. It is thought that colorectal cancers and adenomatous polyps bleed intermittently (Greegor 1971), and this is the basis for recommending that occult blood testing be done on samples taken from three consecutive bowel movements. Blood, if present, is also not homogeneously distributed throughout a stool and, for this reason, it is recommended that two specimens be taken from different parts of the stool for each test. The ingestion of 750 mg or more of vitamin C has been associated with false negatives, apparently by interfering with the test reaction. Several maneuvers have been considered to verify the validity of a test that is thought to be falsely positive. In such cases, it would be economically more reasonable to do a second three-sample test before ordering a full workup of sigmoidoscopy, barium enema and possible colonoscopy. If this is done, dietary restrictions of no red meat or peroxidase-containing vegetables or fruits should be followed for three days prior to, and during, the days of testing. It should also be determined whether aspirin or cimetidine are being taken by the subject, since these both may lead to false positives.

To verify a test which is thought to be falsely negative, the test might also be rerun after putting the patient on a diet high in roughage, which is thought to encourage bleeding by polyps and tumors. Another possibility is to retest for fecal occult blood by using one of the newly developed tests based on antisera to human hemoglobin. These are more sensitive, specific and expensive than the guaiac-based test, although less expensive than a diagnostic workup.

In general, however, the rates of false positive and false negative responses are thought to be low enough to allow serious consideration of guaiac-based testing for fecal occult blood as a mass screening procedure.

It is largely due to a general recognition that other methodologies have too many limitations, that intensive efforts have been mounted to definitively evaluate the testing for occult fecal blood as a mass screen for colorectal cancer. Several large, controlled, prospective studies have been initiated, and reports of their preliminary findings have been published (Gilbertsen et al 1980; Winawer et al 1980). Values of 80% sensitivity, 98% specificity and 75% compliance have been estimated from these studies (Fletcher and Dauphinee 1981). In one of these trials (Winawer et al 1980), about half of 22,000 patients ages 40 years or more were screened for fecal occult blood by means of a 6-slide test protocol while on a red-meat-free high roughage diet. Virtually all of these screened patients and a similar number of control patients were also examined by sigmoidoscopy. Forty-three cancers were detected with the aid of the occult blood test and these had more favorable clinical staging (65% Dukes' A and 13% Dukes' B) than 12 cancers found in the control group. The incidence of colorectal cancer in the screened group was 0.33% in comparison to 0.16% in the control group. This frequency is similar to what has been reported in many uncontrolled studies which, despite a wide variety of protocols, were remarkably similar in discovering colorectal cancer at a rate of 1 or 2 per thousand patients screened (Diehl 1981).

The compliance rate of 74% reported in the controlled study is reasonably reassuring, but as a point of comparison in several less controlled studies it was found that as many as 60%-70% of individuals invited to be screened declined the invitation, and of those that entered the studies, 70%-78% complied by sending the test slides to their physicians (Million R et al 1982; Morrow et al 1982). It was noted by Morrow and his colleagues that noncompliers were, in comparison to compliers,, more elderly, had poorer eyesight, and were less likely to be married, have a family physician or have used Hemoccult slides previously.

These observations concerning acceptance and compliance suggest that there may be room for improvement of the test method as concerns ease of use or esthetic aspects of the conventional Hemoccult test.

EARLY DETECTOR - A NEW, EASIER IN-HOME OCCULT BLOOD TEST

A new guaiac-based test which provides just such improvements has been developed. The procedure is simple, more acceptable to patients and easy to perform in the privacy of the home. Rather than using guaiac-impregnated filter paper, this test uses specially-prepared paper tissue very much like ordinary toilet paper. It differs from toilet paper in that it has two test spots (one treated with hemoglobin and one not) which are used to determine the internal validity of the test. Unlike the cumbersome stick method, the patient takes a fecal sample by the simple means of a gentle patting action (actually just touching the pad gently to their anus). This simplified and esthetically more pleasing collection procedure is permitted by the fact that a method of manufacturing a chemically stable solution of guaiac and peroxidase has been devised. This solution is simply prepared for use by adding a tablet of stabilized guaiac resin to a dispensing bottle containing alcohol and hydrogen peroxide. The solution is ready to use one hour after it has been prepared and then has a shelf-life of four months.

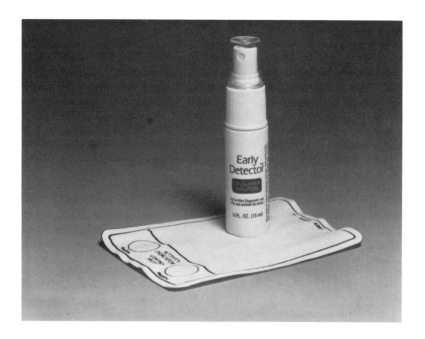

Once the fecal sample has been taken, in this simple manner and for the first time without having to reach into the toilet bowl or bedpan with a wooden stick, the developing solution is sprayed on the sample and the test spots. The development of blue color on the fecal smear within 60 seconds constitutes a positive test.

Obviously, this procedure has some distinct benefits over the conventional guaiac slide tests. First, the blue color of a positive test is directly visible. It is not viewed through the gray transluscence of wet filter paper. Second, the sample size is larger since the specimen on the paper pad is equivalent to two Hemoccult squares. Third, the test is clean and esthetically elegant in comparison to previous methods. After the test is performed, with no need of picking samples from a stool with an applicator, the test pad is simply flushed down the toilet. There is no soiled applicator to be disposed of. There is no storage of slides in the refrigerator and no altered sensitivity due to drying or rehydration.

It seems likely that this test may significantly increase the acceptability and compliance as concerns screening for fecal occult blood.

It is clear that screening for fecal occult blood will usefully shift the detection of colorectal tumors from the excessive proportion of Dukes' C stages toward the more successfully treatable Dukes' A stage. My own response to a patient with a positive occult blood test may be of interest. After checking first to see if there are obvious hemorrhoids or other perianal disease, I do a sigmoidoscopy. However, this is an unprepped sigmoidoscopy which allows me to see if there is any blood in the stool above the anal canal. If blood is present, I proceed directly to colonoscopy. If blood is not present, I do not continue the evaluation unless other signs or symptoms suggest otherwise or unless occult bleeding persists.

The American Cancer Society currently recommends that a woman should perform self-examination of the breast once a month, beginning at age 20; and that men and women both should do occult blood testing only once a year, beginning at age 50! I don't understand this discrepancy. It cannot be due to any substantial difference between the biology of breast cancers and colorectal cancers. Possibly it reflects a distaste for taking stool samples from the toilet bowl with a little stick. Whatever the reason, the dramatic differences between the survivability of patients after resection of localized colorectal cancer as compared to the excessive mortality seen in symptomatic patients warrants serious rethinking of these recommendations.

SUMMARY

For the very first time, an occult blood test has been designed to conform to convenient and natural bathroom habits. For the very first time, we therefore expect the general public to agree willingly to participate in occult blood testing. For the very first time, we expect Early Detector to successfully screen the general public, so that survival rates from colon and rectal cancer may show a significant improvement in the next decade.

REFERENCES

Gilbertsen VA, MacHugh R, Schuman L et al (1980). The earlier detection of colorectal cancers. A preliminary report of the results of the occult blood study. Cancer 45:2899.

Greegor DH (1971). Occult blood testing for detection of asymtomatic colon cancer. Cancer 28:131-134.

Hertz REL, Deddish MR, Day E (1960). Value of periodic examinations in detecting cancer of the rectum and colon. Postgrad Med 27:290.

Kristein MM (1980). The economics of screening for colorectal cancer. Soc Sci Med 14C:275.

Levin DL (1974). "Cancer Rates and Risks," HEW Publication No. (NIH)79:691, 2nd ed, Bethesda, MD, National Inst of Health.

Million R, Howarth J, Turnberg E et al (1982). Faecal occult blood testing for colorectal cancer in general practice. The Practitioner 226:659-663.

Morrow GH, Way J, Hoagland AC, Cooper R (1982). Patient compliance with self-directed Hemoccult testing. Preventive Medicine 11:512-520.

Murphy GP (1977). "Short-term Patient Care Evaluation of Cancer of the Colon". Commission on Cancer, Chicago, Am Coll Surgeons.

Ostrow JD, Mulvaney CA, Hansell JR et al (1973). Sensitivity and reproducibility of chemial tests for fecal occult blood with the emphasis on false positive reaction. Am J Dig Dis 18:930.

Silverberg E (1984). Cancer statistics. CA 34:7.

Songster CL, Barrows GH, Jarritt DD (1980). Immunochemical detection of fecal occult blood - the fecal smear punch disc test! A new non-invasive screening test for colorectal cancer. Cancer 45 (5 suppl):1099-1102.

Stroehlein JR, Fairbanks VF, McGill DB et al (1976). Hemoccult detection of fecal occult blood quantitated by radioassay. Dig Dis 21:841-844.

Walsh TH, Spiro M (1981). How accurately do we diagnose tumors at the rectosigmoid junction? The Practitioner 225:1317.

Winawer SJ (1984). Colorectal cancer can be prevented; 100,000 lives can be saved annually with early detection and treatment. Am J Proctology Gastroenterology and Colon and Rectal Surgery 22-34.

Winawer SJ, Andrews M, Flehinger B et al (1980). Progress report on controlled trial of fecal occult blood testing for the detection of colorectal neoplasia. Cancer 45:2959

Carcinoma of the Large Bowel and Its Precursors, pages 77–90
© 1985 Alan R. Liss, Inc.

CANCER AND DYSPLASIA IN ULCERATIVE COLITIS:
AN INSOLUBLE PROBLEM?

Robert H. Riddell, M.D.
Professor of Pathology
McMaster University Medical Centre
Hamilton, Ontario, CANADA L8N 3Z5

Whether used by pathologists or clinicians, the term 'dysplasia' tends to evoke a sense of frustration which in part stems from a failure to understand the underlying concepts, the morphological appearance, the clinical significance and how each is open to misinterpretation. There is also concern that dysplasia is being missed due to its relative infrequency in clinical practice (Yardley JH, Ransohoff DF, Riddell RH, Goldman H 1983). There may also be frustration because of the uncertainty as to how dysplasia should best be managed, for is there really a "best" time to carry out colectomy? In the eyes of many the ideal time to carry out colectomy is when a small focus of invasive carcinoma is found in the resected specimen that is limited to the submucosa. The clinician then feels that colectomy was not recommended prematurely while the patient can be told that the disease was caught 'just in time' and is almost certainly cured. While such 'ideal' clinical situations do exist, they usually do not reflect the reality of an anxious clinician, pathologist and patient all wondering whether they are recommending the most appropriate therapy at the most appropriate time and weighing the risks of a clinically inapparent but potentially lethal tumor already being present against the operative morbidity and mortality - i.e., the short term risk against the long term benefits.

THE CONCEPT OF DYSPLASIA:

This is based on the assumption that invasive

carcinomas do not arise "de novo" but from a preceding epithelial abnormality that is morphologically recognizable. Such a sequence has been demonstrated in a variety of human organ systems, particularly squamous carcinoma of the uterine cervix, but also in the large bowel where there is ample evidence to support the adenoma-carcinoma sequence. This is derived not only from the literature (Yardley JH et al 1983), but also from a wealth of individual colonoscopic experience, for adenomas containing foci of invasive adenocarcinoma are relatively frequent. The fact that adenomas are by definition dysplastic, but well circumscribed nodules of dysplasia, confirms the essential morphologic similarity between dysplasia in inflammatory bowel disease and adenomas.

A further point of similarity between adenomas and dysplasia in colitis is the manner in which both give rise to invasive carcinoma. Carcinoma arising in an adenoma frequently does so from severely dysplastic crypts, or in-situ carcinoma, but this is not always the case. Indeed in Muto's classic study about 1/3 of the invasive carcinomas arose from adenomas showing only mild dysplasia (Muto T, Bussey HJR, Morson BC 1975). Adenomas do not need to go through the full sequence of changes from mild to moderate to severe (or low grade to high grade) dysplasia culminating in in-situ and finally invasive carcinoma, the fact that they are adenomas provides all of the required potential to invade. However, the more severe the dysplasia, the more likely is that potential to be realized. The same is also true of dysplasia in colitis in that once the same morphological changes (dysplasia) are present in a patient with colitis there is the potential for invasion to occur. Similarly in-situ carcinoma is not required for invasion to occur although it may certainly be present. The clinical significant of this concept is that if one waits until in situ carcinoma develops before recommending colectomy, there is likely to be a high incidence of associated invasive adenocarcinoma; in fact in situ carcinoma without an associated invasive adenocarcinoma is extremely uncommon.

PROBLEMS ASSOCIATED WITH DYSPLASIA IN ULCERATIVE COLITIS:

One of the major problems confronting the management of patients with longstanding ulcerative colitis has been the lack of uniform terminology, definitions and a system of classification. As a result it has been impossible to compare papers from the literature: this has caused considerable confusion. Much of this has stemmed from the failure to separate or even recognize typical reparative changes and distinguish them from neoplastic proliferation, errors that might lead to inappropriate treatment. These problems should no longer cause the same degree of confusion since the publication of a standardized classification of dysplasia in inflammatory bowel disease, a study in which a group of pathologists interested in this subject engaged in several exchanges of slides (Riddell RH et al 1983).

Definition of Dysplasia

The literature uses a variety of terms for epithelial abnormalities which often reflect not only neoplastic but also reparative (regenerative) changes without distinguishing between them. One reason for this is that regenerative changes are relatively poorly described. The situation is clearly simplified if the definition of dysplasia is restricted entirely to an <u>unequivocally neoplastic</u> proliferation. All regenerative or even doubtful epithelial proliferations should be excluded from this definition (Riddell RH et al 1983). A very good analogy can be made with villous adenomas, in which the dysplastic mucosa of the adenoma gives rise directly to an occult invasive carcinoma that may only be found on resection.

Morphological Differences in the Pathogenesis of Dysplasia in Ulcerative Colitis and Adenomas

Adenomas and dysplasia in ulcerative colitis are by definition frequently indistinguishable morphologically, both representing an unequivocally neoplastic proliferation, why then bother to distinguish between them? The reasons are threefold:

(a) Pathogenesis: The earliest phase in the formation of adenomas - namely, a single neoplastic (or dysplastic) crypt - is readily demonstrable in familial adenomatous polyposis coli; the difference between such a crypt and the adjacent crypts is obvious. It is essentially an all-or-none phenomenon. Although similar changes may be seen in colitis, dysplasia is frequently part of a spectrum of changes rather than the all-or-none changes seen in adenomas. Implicit in any spectrum of changes is the fact that although comparisons between different parts reveal obvious differences, all divisions within the spectrum are necessarily arbitrary and subjective. Similarly, while major differences in the spectrum may well be significant, minor discrepancies may be virtually irrelevant.

(b) Implications: Stated simply, the diagnosis of an adenoma whether in a colitic or a non-colitic, may lead to the literal interpretation that a typical adenoma has been biopsied, whereas in a colitic the biopsy may actually have come from the surface of an invasive carcinoma that was not recognized endoscopically, the so-called "dyspla-sia-associated lesion or mass" (DALM) (Blackstone MO, Riddell RH, Rogers BHG, Levin B 1981). In an identical clinical setting the diagnosis of "dysplasia" as opposed to "adenoma," immediately serves as an alert that either a DALM has been biopsied or that the patient is in a parti-cularly high risk group of having an occult invasive carcinoma elsewhere in the large bowel.

(c) Adenomas in colitis: Many patients with UC are in the age range where they may be expected to develop adenomas; further, in some colitics lesions indistinguish-able from tubular adenomas (adenomatous polyps) are found. Whether these are of any greater significance than adenomas found in the non-colitic population is not know, but it seems likely that this would be the case in patients generally regarded as outside this range - i.e., less than about 45 years old (Riddell RH 1980). These lesions are relatively common, particularly in older patients with UC but complete endoscopic polypectomy is probably adequate. In young patients, however, although treatment may be along similar lines, it is clearly worrying and close follow-up is necessary to ensure that other similar lesions, or carcinomas, are not present elsewhere. Thus, whether the development of such lesions in colitics, particularly in younger patients, is a marker of those more likely to develop carcinomas, as seems likely, is actually unknown.

THE SPECTRUM AND SIGNIFICANCE OF MUCOSAL CHANGES FOUND

In examining biopsies from patients at risk major divisions within the spectrum need to be made because they are of clinical significance. Thus biopsies can be divided into those that are unequivocally neoplastic (positive for dysplasia), those which are unequivocally negative for dysplasia, included in which are typical quiescent, active or resolving colitis including typical reparative changes. The mid-part of the spectrum - namely, those not falling into either of these two categories - are indefinite for dysplasia. Included in this category are those patients whose epithelium may be progressing through the spectrum and which may ultimately terminate in dysplasia, those with exuberant reparative processes which are beyond those acceptable as falling within the norm and other types of epithelial prolifera- tion not readily classifiable (Riddell RH et al 1983).

The clinical value of this classification is that it can be combined with the options for patient management (repeated colonoscopy at the usual time interval, repeated colonoscopy at a shorter time interval, polypectomy) as shown in Table 1. As can be seen from this Table the vast majority of patients whose biopsies are negative as well as those with slightly exuberant changes thought most likely to be the result of inflammation will be re- colonoscoped at the appropriate regular clinical interval, usually annually. Those with more worrisome changes (indefinite for dysplasia - unknown and indefinite for dysplasia - probably positive) will undergo repeat colonoscopy with multiple biopsies at a much shorter interval of time. As discussed above, patients who have unequivocal dysplasia are at significant risk from either having or developing invasive carcinoma, but the extent of this risk is unknown because of lack of appropriate clinical data.

MANAGEMENT OF DYSPLASIA

The management of "adenomas", and the possibility of their being treated only by local complete excision, has been discussed above. Patients with dysplasia on biopsy, as defined above, are clearly already at risk of having an invasive carcinoma. The major question in this group of

TABLE 1:   Provisional Schema of Patient Management Related
           to Classification of Dysplasia

Biopsy Classification	Implications for Patient Management
Negative Normal Mucosa Inactive (quiescent) colitis Active colitis Indefinite Probably negative	Continue regular follow-up
Unknown Probably positive	Institute short-interval follow-up
Positive Low-grade dysplasia	Institute short-interval follow-up or Consider colectomy, especially with gross lesion, after dysplasia is confirmed.
High-grade dysplasia	Consider colectomy after dysplasia is confirmed.

patients is whether the risk is high enough for them to consider undergoing proctocolectomy. Apart from the dysplasia itself, there are a variety of other factors that affect the likelihood of the patient having an underlying carcinoma. These are whether the dysplasia is high grade or low grade, whether the dysplastic biopsies were obtained from a mucosal abnormality (mass or lesion).

(a) Dysplastic biopsy taken from an endoscopically irregular lesion: This is particularly important because the presence of an endoscopic abnormality from which a dysplastic biopsy is obtained is highly significant, there being a very high probability that this represents the superficial part of an invasive adenoma (Blackstone, Riddell, Rogers, Levin 1981). Such lesions should always therefore be considered clinically to be invasive carcinomas until proven otherwise and managed appropriately. In most cases the appropriate management is surgical resection. It cannot be overemphasized that such carcinomas may show only low grade dysplasia on biopsies; in some carcinomas the mucosa from which the carcinoma is clearly arising sometimes shows only epithelium indefinite for dysplasia, a source of particular frustration.

(b) The significance of dysplasia being found on a first, as opposed to a subsequent, colonoscopy is the increased likelihood of there being an associated carcinoma should colectomy be carried out at this stage with or without an endoscopic abnormality. In patients who have undergone several surveillance colonoscopies all of which have yielded biopsies negative for dysplasia, the finding in a subsequent colonoscopy of dysplasia suggests that it has most likely developed in the more recent past, although because of the sampling problems involved this can never be adequately documented. However, if found at the first colonoscopy it is more likely that the changes have been present for a longer period of time and therefore are more likely to have undergone malignant transformation. Some think that this distinction is so important that the first colonoscopy is called "diagnostic" and subsequent colonoscopies "surveillance" (Fuson et al 1980).

(c) The grade of dysplasia is important in that high grade dysplasia is almost certainly much more likely to be associated with an invasive carcinoma than low grade dysplasia. However, the fact that low grade dysplasia has

a significant association with invasive carcinoma implies
that unexpected carcinomas can always be expected, albeit
in a small number of patients, whenever low grade dysplasia is present.

Early Cancer Detection or Cancer Prevention

One of the major difficulties in the follow-up of
patients with diseases like colitis at risk from developing carcinoma is what the purpose of the colonoscopy
should be and also its end-point. There are really only
two options - namely to detect carcinoma at the earliest
possible time clinically or to attempt to prevent the
development of invasive carcinoma - but their significance
is very different. The former implies a policy of waiting
until a carcinoma develops endoscopically, possibly as a
DALM, at which time colectomy would be recommended This
policy would result in a relatively high number of
associated carcinomas but the clinical hope would be that
these would be relatively "early" and would be cured by
resection. The advantage of this policy is that
resections in which no carcinoma was found would be
relatively few. The obvious disadvantage of this policy
is that in many patients the carcinoma would already
either have invaded through the entire thickness of the
muscularis propria or have lymph node metastases (or
worse) so that the chances of a curative resection being
carried out are relatively low.

In contrast, the policy of cancer prevention is one
that can be managed at a variety of levels. One extreme
of this is the policy of prophylactic proctocolectomy that
was so popular in the 1960's. However, while the chance
of an invasive carcinoma being found was low and the
chance of a subsequent carcinoma developing in the large
bowel was removed, the limiting factor in the risk vs.
benefit equation became the operative morbidity and
mortality. Although the risk of finding a curable cancer
was similar to the operative mortality, death occurred
much sooner in the surgical group. These findings and the
failure of patients to accept colectomy ultimately lead to
the abandonment of this policy.

AT WHAT POINT SHOULD COLECTOMY BE ADVISED?

If a tangible fact such as a 10-year history of extensive colitis is not to be the endpoint in the decision for proctocolectomy, then what should the endpoint be? As discussed above, if any grade of dysplasia is found associated with an endoscopic lesion or mass, particularly if found at the first colonoscopy then colectomy is indicated in view of the high risk of the lesion actually being a carcinoma. If high grade dysplasia without an endoscopic irregularity is the endpoint then the literature, difficult as it is to interpret, suggests that probably about one-third to two-thirds of these patients will already have an invasive carcinoma (Hulten, Kewenter, Ahren 1972; van Heerden, Beart 1980; Warren, Sommers 1949; Dawson Pryse-Davies 1959; Cook, Goligher 1975; Fenoglio, Pascal 1973; Gewertz, Dent, Appelman 1979; Nugent FW et al 1979; Yardley, Keren 1974; Kewenter, Hulten, Ahren 1982). If the finding of high grade dysplasia is too late, then is low grade dysplasia an acceptable endpoint? Such patients would clearly already be at risk of having a carcinoma but this is probably much lower than those with high grade dysplasia and probably in the vicinity of 10% although hard data is again lacking. In many ways this makes the most sense in that, by definition, low grade dysplasia is already capable of giving rise directly to an invasive carcinoma. Within the group of patients with UC at risk of developing cancer, these patients have demonstrated the ability of their large bowel mucosa to undergo neoplastic transformation. If one is therefore to negotiate the difficult course between Scylla and Charybdis then this would be the most appropriate time to undergo colectomy.

In Table 1 there is only one other option, which is to consider colectomy at the stage of 'indefinite for dysplasia'. This would lower the chances of finding an incidental carcinoma further, probably to the region of less than 3% but may also include the majority of patients being followed, a situation not far removed from prophylactic colectomy after 10 years of disease, except that for some patients colectomy may be postponed for an undefined length of time.

In summary, the current theoretically "best" time to carry out proctocolectomy is at the stage of low grade dysplasia. However it has to be stressed that because reproducibility is not absolute, even between interested pathologists, that it is essential that the diagnosis is confirmed before colectomy is carried out. This can be either by letting a further pathologist with an interest in the disease and familiar with this system of classification review the slides, or by repeating the biopsies, or both. However, because dysplasia is frequently a focal lesion, repeat colonoscopy may fail to find the dysplastic area, possibly leading to an assumption that the dysplasia has 'regressed' or 'disappeared'. Conversely the insistence on obtaining repeated dysplastic biopsies will reduce the likelihood of colectomy being carried out for biopsies that have been misinterpreted as being positive for dysplasia (i.e., false positives). Obviously the greater the degree of certainty about the diagnosis, the less likely the risk of carrying out an unnecessary colectomy.

RISK OF DEVELOPING DYSPLASIA

It is clear that long-term management of patients in this high risk group is ultimately dependent upon the likelihood of their developing dysplasia. From the literature it is apparent that the risk of developing carcinoma in ulcerative colitis varies considerably from one part of the world to another; areas like Israel having a very low incidence (Gilat et al 1974); while areas like Chicago appear to have a much greater incidence. In a study at the University of Chicago the cumulative proportion of patients developing high grade dysplasia was found to be 7% at 20 years, 16% at 30 years, and 25% at 37 years. Low grade dysplasia developed in 30% at 20 years, 60% at 30 years, and 90% at 37 years (Hanover, Riddell, Kirsner, Levin 1983). These figures are very disconcerting because they imply that most patients with longstanding ulcerative colitis will ultimately develop dysplasia and (if the guidelines used above are followed) of undergoing proctocolectomy. However, these figures have yet to be confirmed although, should they prove to be accurate, one will be left in a similar position to that of the 1960's in knowing that most patients may well eventually come to colectomy. The only important factor would therefore be in the timing of this operation.

RISK OF DEVELOPING CARCINOMA DESPITE REGULAR FOLLOW-UP

It seems likely that in UC the only method of treatment that is likely to result in a virtual absence of carcinomas is that of early prophylactic proctocolectomy. Any other means of follow-up will inevitably be associated with a definite risk of carcinoma. If the classification of dysplasia as suggested here is used, then the further along this spectrum one progresses, the more likely will be the risk of a carcinoma developing. There are, however, other reasons for suggesting that occasionally carcinomas may prove lethal irrespective of how frequently or well colonoscopy is carried out.

(a) Carcinomas in ulcerative colitis are frequently small, plaque-like or finely nodular or sometimes not even raised above the adjacent mucosa. They may therefore escape clinical detection. In this manner they clearly bear some resemblance to early gastric carcinoma type Ib.

(b) If one waits for the development of dysplasia then, by definition, some of the dysplastic lesions will prove to be invasive carcinomas on resection.

(c) Occasional carcinomas are found which appear to be arising from mucosa which is less far along the morphological spectrum than conventional low grade dysplasia - i.e., occasionally carcinomas appear to develop from mucosa that is indefinite for dysplasia (Riddell, in press). Fortunately, these are relatively uncommon but they do reflect a relative inability to distinguish all forms of neoplastic proliferation. On some occasions such carcinomas may form mucin pools and therefore be colloid carcinomas, but because of the lack of dysplasia within either the overlying epithelium or the tumor itself, it may be misdiagnosed as colitis cystica profunda.

(d) Some patients will develop carcinoma because they refuse to undergo colectomy when this is recommended or simply fail to return for surveillance colonoscopies. In this regard it is essential for patients moving away to continue surveillance, a change in which the patient's physician should actively participate.

For all of these reasons it seems unlikely that, until

better markers are found we will be able to completely prevent the development of invasive carcinoma. Nevertheless, this apparent air of gloom must be counterbalanced by the fact that most large surveillance programs are surprisingly successful in preventing patients from developing lethal tumors.

MARKERS FOR DYSPLASIA

A variety of markers have been suggested for detecting dysplastic mucosa but so far none of these appears of value. Carcino-embryonic antigen (CEA) seems to be valueless as it is present in both regenerative and neoplastic mucosa. The high iron diamine stain to detect sulfated mucopolysaccharides seems completely insensitive (Riddell - unpublished observations). The presence of unusual lectins such as peanut agglutinin (PNA) may be of value (Boland, Lance, Levin, Riddell, Kim in press), but are also unproven. One study looking at the DNA content of epithelial nuclei in UC found these changes unhelpful in distinguishing regenerative from dysplastic mucosa (Hammerberg, Slezak, Tribukait 1984). To date, therefore, there is still no substitution for regular light microscopy.

POINTERS FOR THE FUTURE

Much has still to be learned regarding the management of patients with longstanding extensive UC. All patients should at least be in some form of surveillance program looking for either dysplasia or "early" carcinoma (usually both). The timing of the recommendations for colectomy is usually based not only on the presence or absence of dysplasia but also the activity of the disease, how well the patient copes with it or responds to therapy, worries about the ability to have or father children, the attitudes and competence of all involved in the decision for colectomy. In most large centers this complex situation is handled surprisingly well as judged by the relatively few patients in surveillance programs dying of carcinoma. Nevertheless this is not always the case. It is clear that until relatively specific markers for either dysplasia or minimally invasive carcinoma are developed, that the decision to recommend colectomy will still depend on too many variables.

The risk of invasive carcinoma being present when low grade or high grade dysplasia, or even epithelium indefinite for dysplasia is found on biopsy both with and without an endoscopic abnormality, needs to be accurately documented whether at the first or subsequent colonoscopy. The effect of geographic differences in incidence also needs consideration. Such studies are best carried out prospectively. We will then be in a position to advise our patients of their risk of having a carcinoma based on sound data. In doing so we may have at least found partial solution to this problem.

REFERENCES

Blackstone MO, Riddell RH, Rogers BHG, Levin B (1981). Dysplasia-associated lesion or mass (DALM) detected by colonoscopy in longstanding ulcerative colitis: an indication for colectomy. Gastroenterology 80:366-374.

Boland CR, Lance P, Levin B, Riddell RH, Kim YS. Gut (in press).

Cook MG, Goligher JC (1975). Carcinoma and epithelial dysplasia complicating ulcerative colitis. Gastroenterology 68:1127-1136.

Dawson IMP, Pryse-Davies J (1959). The development of carcinoma of the large intestine in ulcerative colitis. Br J Surg 47:113-128.

Fenoglio CM, Pascal RR (1973). Adenomatous epithelium, intraepithelial anaplasia, and invasive carcinoma in ulcerative colitis. Am J Dig Dis 18:556-562.

Fuson JA, Farmer RG, Hawk WA, Sullivan BH (1980). Endoscopic surveillance for cancer in chronic ulcerative colitis. Am J Gastroenterol 73:120-126.

Gewertz BL, Dent TL, Appelman HD (1976). Implications of precancerous rectal biopsy in patients with inflammatory bowel disease. Arch Surg 111:326-329.

Gilat T, Zemishlany Z, Ribak J, Benaroya Y, Lilos P (1974). Ulcerative colitis in the Jewish population of Tel Aviv Yafo. II. Rarity of malignant degeneration. Gastroenterology 67:933-938.

Hammarberg C, Slezak P, Tribukait B (1984). Early detection of malignancy in UC: A Flow-Cytometric DNA Study. Cancer 53(2):291-295.

Hanauer SB, Riddell RH, Kirsner JB, Levin B (1983). Life-table analysis of onset of dysplasia in chronic ulcerative colitis (CUC). Gastroenterology (Abstract)84:1181.

Hulten L, Kewenter J, Ahren C (1972). Precancer and carcinoma in chronic ulcerative colitis: a histopathological and clinical investigation. Scand J Gastroenterol 7:663-669.

Kewenter J, Hulten L, Ahren C (1982). The occurrence of severe epithelial dysplasia and its bearing on treatment of longstanding ulcerative colitis. Ann Surg 195:209-213.

Muto T, Bussey HJR, Morson BC (1975). The evolution of cancer of the colon and rectum. Cancer 36:2251-2270.

Nugent FW, Haggitt RC, Colcher H, Kutteruf GC (1979). Malignant potential of chronic ulcerative colitis: preliminary report. Gastroenterology 76:1-5.

Riddell RH (1980). Dysplasia in inflammatory bowel disease. Clinics in Gastroenterol 9:439-458.

Riddell RH, Goldman H, Ransohoff DF, Appleman HD, Fenoglio CM, Haggit RC, Ahren C, Correa P, Hamilton SR, Morson BC, Sommers SC, Yardley JH (1983). Dysplasia in inflammatory bowel disease. Human Pathology 14:931-968.

Riddell RH (in press). Dysplasia and cancer in ulcerative colitis: a soluble problem? Scand J Gastroenterol.

van Heerden JA, Beart RW Jr (1980). Carcinoma of the colon and rectum complicating chronic ulcerative colitis. Dis Colon Rectum 23:155-159.

Warren S, Sommers SC (1949). Pathogenesis of ulcerative colitis. Am J Pathol 25:657-679.

Yardley JH, Ransohoff DF, Riddell RH, Goldman H (1983). Cancer in inflammatory bowel disease: How serious is the problem and what should be done about it? Gastroenterology (Edit) 85:197-200.

Yardley JH, Keren DF (1974). "Precancer" lesions in ulcerative colitis: a retrospective study of rectal biopsy and colectomy specimens. Cancer 34:835-844.

Carcinoma of the Large Bowel and Its Precursors, pages 91–101
© 1985 Alan R. Liss, Inc.

COLORECTAL CANCER IN CROHN'S COLITIS AND OTHER LARGE
INTESTINAL DISEASES: IS THERE A DYSPLASIA-CARCINOMA
SEQUENCE?

Roy G. Shorter, M.D., F R.C.P.. F.A.C.P.
Professor of Medicine and Pathology
Mayo Medical School
Rochester, Minnesota 55905

Although it is established (and accepted) that there
is an increased risk of colorectal cancer in patients in
the U.S.A. or the U.K. who have extensive chronic ulcera-
give colitis (CUC) of long duration (> 10 years) (Thayer,
1980), the magnitude of the risk in Crohn's colitis
remains a somewhat controversial issue. This is due
largely to the fact that until about ten years ago it was
widely held that such patients were not at increased risk
of large bowel cancer, despite the lack of data to support
such a conclusion, and there appears to be some lingering
reluctance to abandon this view (Butt, Lennard-Jones,
Ritchie 1980) even though there is good information to the
contrary. The latter has been provided by three major
reports from the U.S.A. and the U.K. (Weedon, Shorter,
Ilstrup, Huizenga, Taylor 1973; Gyde, Prior, Macartney,
Thompson, Waterhouse, Allan 1980; Greenstein, Sachar,
Smith, Janowitz, Aufses 1980), in the earliest of which
Shorter's group studied 449 patients with Crohn's disease
(CD) who were 21 years of age or younger when first seen
at the Mayo Clinic between 1919 and 1965 (Weedon, Shorter,
Ilstrup, Huizenga, Taylor, 1973). Sixty-three percent
were males, 26 percent were Jewish, all were white, all
were residents of North America, except for one Austra-
lian, and the mean age at the onset of symptoms of CD was
14.9 years. The duration of symptoms prior to their first
attendance at the Mayo Clinic averaged 2.5 years in those
first seen before 1953, and 1.8 years in those first seen
after 1953. At the time of presentation, 21 percent had
Crohn's enteritis, 58 percent had enterocolitis and 21
percent had colitis. Four hundred and forty-two (98.4

percent) were followed up either to their death or to October 31, 1972; for the seven in whom follow-up was incomplete, information was obtained for part of the period and they were considered "withdrawn alive" at the time either of their last attendance at the Mayo Clinic or their last consultation with a local physician. Acceptance of a diagnosis of supervening cancer demanded pathological confirmation both of the tumor and the coexistence of CD, and in calculating survival rates and the risk of cancer, life-table methods were used. In the analysis of the risk of malignancy, three groups were regarded as "withdrawn" for part of the time, in keeping with actuarial methods. These included the seven individuals for whom complete follow-up data were not available, those who died without evidence of cancer and who were withdrawn as of the date of death, and those treated by total proctocolectomy for enterocolitis or colitis. The latter were considered withdrawn as of the date on which the removal of all the colon and rectum was completed, provided that the resected specimen was free of cancer. During the course of their disease, 109 of the patients had total proctocolectomy, either as a staged or single procedure, while 144 had total colectomy, either staged or as a single procedure, with preservation of the rectum. The expected number of cases of cancer of the large intestine was calculated by applying the combined age-specific, sex-specific and decade-specific incidence rates for cancer of the colon and rectum in the population of Connecticut to the actuarial estimates of the age-specific, sex-specific and decade-specific person-years lived by the 449 patients with Crohn's disease.

Cancer was found in 12 patients at some time after their first attendance at the Mayo Clinic. The primary site was in the colon in seven, in the rectum in one, and elsewhere in the other four (jejunum, 1; breast, 1; ovary, 1; undetermined, 1). Of the seven colonic cancers, the ascending colon was the site in five, the transverse colon in one, and the descending colon in the other. The shortest period between the onset of symptoms of CD and the diagnosis of colonorectal cancer was seven years, and the longest was 45 years. Five of the eight with large bowel cancer had enterocolitis, while the other three had extensive colitis. Each of the cancers occurred in bowel grossly involved by CD and five died as a direct result of the tumors.

Although the 10-year probability of remaining cancer free was 99.7 percent and the 20-year probability was 97.2 percent, an impressive finding was the youth of six of the eight patients when they were found to have large intestinal cancer (21, 23, 23, 28, 37, 37, 45 and 55 years). Furthermore, calculation of the expected incidence of carcinoma of the large bowel showed that the finding of eight cases of large intestinal cancer was approximately 20 times greater than expected (0.3 cases; P<0.001), assuming a distribution as a Poisson variable. The risk was even more striking if the analysis was restricted to the 356 who had colonic involvement by CD. The conclusion that the patients were at increased risk of developing large intestinal cancer was facilitated by the fact that follow-up data were incomplete in only seven. In the life-table analyses it was considered reasonable to assume that for these seven an event in question would have occurred with the same probability as for the rest. However, if these seven "withdrawals" differed from the remainder of the study group, thus leading to biased probability estimates, the small number could not have modified the conclusion about the risk of cancer of the large bowel.

One possible bias was recognized, namely the withdrawal, at the time of completion of proctocolectomy, of those who underwent either total or staged proctocolectomy for treatment of their CD, because on its completion they were no longer at risk of large-bowel cancer. However, in most instances the proctocolectomy was done because of disease severity and/or chronicity, so it is possible that without operation the incidence of cancer would have been higher in these patients than in the rest, and it seems unlikely that it would have been lower.

In summary, this study indicated (1) that those in the U.S.A. with an onset of CD in childhood and long-standing, extensive colonic involvement are at an approximately twenty-fold increased risk of developing carcinoma of the large bowel; (2) that such cancers tend to occur at a relatively young age; (3) that a very large series would be necessary to determine in the U.S.A. the risk of primary cancer of the small bowel in CD; (4) that in CD there is no increased risk of developing extraintestinal primary malignancies.

The Cancer Epidemiology Research Unit in Birmingham, England also published a report on malignancy complicating CD in which the study group consisted of 513 individuals with CD (males:females = 1:1) who were under long-term review between 1944 and December 31, 1976 (Gyde, Prior, Macartney, Thompson, Waterhouse, Allan 1980). However, no details of its ethnic composition were provided. In contrast to Weedon's study, this series was not restricted to those with an onset of CD in childhood, and all but two were over 21 years old when they developed the first recognizable symptoms of CD; the mean age at the onset of these symptoms was approximately 29 years and their mean duration prior to diagnosis was 2.5 years. Nearly 50 percent of the study group had gross disease in the ileum (with or without disease in the right side of the colon) while 34 percent had extensive colonic disease with or without terminal ileal involvement. During the period of observation, panproctocolectomy was carried out in 88 patients, 50 were treated by colectomy and ileorectal anastomosis, and nine patients were lost to follow-up. Since all the group resided in the West Midlands Region of England, the cancer incidence rates for that area were used in evluating the cancer risks.

Thirty-one malignant tumors were found during the observation period, a number which significantly exceeded the expected value of 19. The excess was contributed by tumors of the gastrointestinal (GI) tract, two of which occurred in by-passed intestinal loops. Nine patients developed cancer of the large bowel (sites not listed); this represented a four-fold increased risk which was almost doubled when the analysis was limited to those with extensive colonic CD. At the time of the diagnosis of large-bowel carcinoma the patients' ages ranged from 19 to 55 years and the duration of symptoms of CD from nine to 36 years. However, those without extensive Crohn's colitis showed no increased incidence of large intestinal cancer. Lastly, the numbers of primary tumors at extraintestinal sites did not exceed the expected values.

As a postscriptum, the authors mentioned that two more upper GI cancers and three additional colonic carcinomas were diagnosed during the four years that elapsed between the completion of their study and its publication.

In summary, from this report it can be concluded (1)

that patients in the U.K. with CD are at increased risk of certain gastrointestinal carcinomas, especially colonic cancer (at least fourfold) when the colon has been extensively involved by long-standing disease (>9 years). Although a long duration of the CD is a significant antecedent factor, the increased risk is not limited to those with an onset of CD in childhood. Parenthetically, although Gyde, Prior, Macartney, Thompson, Waterhouse, and Allan (1980) stressed that some of the upper gastrointestinal cancers were found in sites which were "uninvolved" by Crohn's disease, electron microscopic studies suggest that ultramicroscopic abnormalities exist diffusely throughout the bowel, even in the absence of gross lesions (Goodman, Skinner, Truelove 1976; Dvorak, Dickersin 1980). (2) That to establish the magnitude of the risk in the U.K. or primary carcinoma of the small bowel in CD would require an extremely large study group.

The third of the major reports in this investigative area is that by Greenstein, Sachar, Smith, Janowitz and Aufses (1980) who studied 579 individuals with CD (male:female=1:1) who were admitted to the Mount Sinai Hospital in New York City in the period 1960 to 1976. The ethnic composition of this series was not described. In approximately 44 percent the gross disease was limited to the small bowel, approxiamtely 44 percent had enterocolitis, while the remainder had colitis; the mean age at the onset of symptoms of CD was 26 years. Thirty neoplasms developed in 28 patients, of which 17 were gastrointestinal in origin, and 13, extraintestinal. Nine cancers occurred in the large bowel (three in surgically excluded loops) but their sites were not listed; however, two developed in areas showing no gross evidence of Crohn's disease. In each of four patients, primary carcinoma of the small bowel was found in a surgically-excluded loop grossly involved by CD. "Pancreaticoduodenal" cancer occurred in one individual and carcinoma of the stomach in another; the primary sites could not be determined for the remaining two tumors classified as "intestinal cancers." In all instances the symptoms of CD had been present 'for years' when the diagnosis of complicating gastrointestinal cancer was made. The investigators concluded that in CD patients in the U.S.A. there is a steadily increasing risk of GI cancer with each decade of follow-up, and that there is a markedly increased risk of large bowel cancer (at least seven-fold). They suggested that the reason why the magnitude of the increased risk of large bowel cancer in their series was less than that found by others (Weedon, Shorter, Ilstrup, Huizenga, Taylor 1973) was because the mean duration of the CD was shorter. The sites of the 13 primary extraintestinal malignancies were very varied and included the breast, urinary bladder, thyroid and skin. Although it is not clear how these observed numbers of extraintestinal tumors compared with expected values, it is apparent that neither these findings nor those of the other two studies (Weedon, Shorter, Ilstrup, Huizenga, Taylor 1973: Gyde, Prior, Macartney, Thompson, Waterhouse, Allan 1980) support earlier contentions that patients with CD are at increased risk of cancer of the pancreas or the biliary tract.

Thus, the New York group extended the information on the risk of large bowel cancer in CD in the U.S.A. by providing data from those with an onset of CD in adult life. Secondly, it stressed that such cancers may occur in sites showing no gross evidence of CD and, thirdly, that surgically excluded loops of bowel may be at particular risk of cancerous change. The series was too small to determine whether CD is associated with an increased risk of primary cancer of the small bowel.

Parenthetically, while for many years it has been widely held that a cancer of the colon complicating chronic ulcerative colitis is "intrinsically" a highly malignant tumor, some data have challenged this and suggest that the prognosis of such tumors is as good (or as poor) as that of colorectal carcinomas in general and is related to the Dukes' classification at the time of resection (Butt, Lennard-Jones, Ritchie 1980; Hughes, Hall, Block 1978; Hulten, Kewenter, Ahren 1972). However, the situation in Crohn's disease is unknown.

At this juncture, some points are worthy of statement or restatement: (1) in the U.S.A or the U.K. individuals of either sex with long-standing (>7 years), extensive Crohn's colitis, regardless of age at its onset, are at increased risk (up to 20 X) of colonic cancer, but it is unknown whether an increased risk exists in such patients in other countries. Although it has been suggested that the risk is less in CD than in long-standing CUC, Thayer (1980) contends that it is similar, and his argument to support this view is more persuasive than those used by others to justify a contrary conclusion. The magnitude of the risk of small intestinal cancer in CD is unknown. (2) It seems that the epithelium in surgically by-passed intestinal loops involved by long-standing CD is particularly liable to cancerous change. Thus, it is fortunate that resection has replaced "bypass" in the surgical treatment of this disease. (3) Because ultrastructural changes have been found in the bowel in CD in the absence of gross lesions, it seems inappropriate now to categorize any part of the GI tract as "uninvolved." This view is supported indirectly by clinical observations that following therapeutic resection of gut grossly involved by CD, the incidence of clinical recrudescence is similar whether wide resection is done to achieve margins free from pathological changes (as judged by light microscopy), or whether the resection is conservative and limited to the macroscopically involved area (Pennington, Hamilton, Bayless, Cameron JL 1980). (4) As in CUC, dysplasia may occur in the colonic epithelium in Crohn's disease at sites separate from concomitant colonic cancer (Riddell, Goldman, Ransohoff, Appelman, Haggitt, Ahren, Correa, Hamilton, Morson, Sommers, Yardley 1983). However, as McManus (1982) concluded, the initially optimistic claims for the significance of certain dysplastic changes to the early detection of colonic cancer in idiopathic inflammatory bowel disease have not been sustained. The problems include a failure clearly to establish the specificities and sensitivities of the various degrees of dysplasia as "markers" of cancer elsewhere in the large bowel. This point will be addressed again later. (5) Although in the U.S.A. and the U.K. an increased risk of colorectal carcinoma exists in long-standing CD of the large bowel, the total number of patients at risk is small, as is the number in which large intestinal cancer will occur (Weedon, Shorter, Ilstrup, Huizenga, Taylor 1973; Gyde, Prior, Macartney, Thompson, Waterhouse, Allan 1980; Greenstein, Sachar, Smith, Janowitz, Aufses 1980). Accordingly, the risk should be kept in perspective and the majority of those with CD need not "run scared." However, for the small subgroup that is at increased risk of large bowel carcinoma, careful supervision seems advisable, including repeated colonoscopoies and biopsy sampling, in collaboration with a gastrointestinal pathologist skilled in interpreting dysplasia. Nevertheless, the early diagnosis of cancer complicating CD is very difficult and it is unknown whether such careful "follow-up" will improve the rate of early diagnosis (i.e., the detection of Dukes' A or B tumors). This point, too, will be considered further later.

Apart from idiopathic inflammatory bowel disease (IBD), patients with certain other large intestinal diseases are at variably increased risk of colorectal cancer, particularly those with familial polyposis (or with Gardner's, Turcot's or Oldfield's syndromes) in whom the malignant potential must be considered as 100% (Bussey, 1980: Kent, Mitros 1983). Lesser degrees of increased risk also exist in certain 'colorectal cancer families', in which the mode of inheritance is not well defined (in contrast to familial polyposis), and those family members who develop such cancers usually have pre-existing colorectal adenomas (Morson, Konishi 1980). Furthermore, the incidence of colorectal cancer in first-degree relatives of individuals in the general population who are undergoing treatment for large bowel cancer is approximately threefold higher than expected; in addition, following partial colonic resection for carcinomas, a patient is at considerable risk of developing another primary colorectal cancer, particularly if adenomatous polyps also were present in the resected bowel (Bussey, Wallace, Morson 1967). In countries in which a high incidence of colorectal cancer exists the incidence of large colorectal adenomatous polyps also is high, in contrast to the state of affairs in countries with a low incidence of large bowel cancer (Morson, Konishi 1980). Thus, in high risk areas of the world, for those patients who do not have familial polyposis but do have adenomatous large bowel polyps the risk of colorectal cancer is increased, particularly if the polyp(s) is large (>2 cm) and of the villous type (Morson, Konishi 1980).

Morson and Konishi (1980) suggested that mucosal epithelial dysplasia is the histological and cytological precursor (sine qua non) of large bowel cancer in patients with colorectal adenomas and in those with IBD, i.e. there is a 'dysplasia-cancer' sequence. They stressed that various grades of severity of dysplasia may coexist in colorectal adenomas (perhaps indicating a transition from a benign to a malignant tumor) and that small areas of severe epithelial dysplasia ('carcinoma in situ') have not been found independently of adenomas or idiopathic inflammatory bowel disease. Accordingly, they concluded that it

is likely that all carcinomas of the large bowel emerge
either by an 'adenoma-dysplasia-cancer' or an 'IBD-
dysplasia-cancer' sequence. However, despite the attract-
iveness of this concept it is 'not proven' by the
available data. For example, small, invasive, ulcerating
carcinomas do occur without evidence of a pre-existing
adenoma (Spratt, Ackerman 1962); Morson and Konishi (1980)
attempt to explain these away by suggesting that such
lesions result from extensive cancerous invasion plus surface ulceration in a pre-existing adenoma, thus resulting
in total replacement of the adenomatous tissue. The limitations of this argument are apparent, and their conten-
tion that if large bowel cancers could arise against a
background of normal mucosa then numerous examples of tiny
independent carcinomas inevitably would have been
reported, might be a non sequitur. Clearly, much further
study of the epidemiology of large intestinal epithelial
dysplasia is needed to test their hypothesis, and so to
evaluate the significance of the finding of such dysplasia
to cancer surveillance. This is underlined by the fact
that only lately has there been any modest concensus on
the nature and classification of the qualitative
dysplastic changes which may occur in the colorectal
epithelium in IBD (Riddell, Goldman, Ransohoff, Appleman,
Fenoglio, Haggitt, Ahren, Correa, Hamilton, Morson,
Sommers, Yardley 1983), and even in this extensive
"exchange-review" of material the level of disagreement
between observers was disappointingly high, so it is
obvious that a quantitative method is sorely needed. As
McManus (1984) pointed out recently, a study in London,
England (Lennard-Jones, Ritchie, Morson, Williams 1983)
involving 186 patients with CUC of more than 10 years'
duration who were subjected to extensive 'cancer surveillance' over a 15-year period, including biopsy eva-
luations for epithelial dysplasia in the large bowel,
showed that severe dysplasia in such mucosal samples does
not imply the inevitability of developing large intestinal
cancer, although its presence may indicate an increased
risk of unknown magnitude. While the latter suggestion
seems reasonable, it is impossible currently to conclude
that cancer of the large bowel only emerges from a
dysplasia-cancer sequence. Although this may be true, the
proof is lacking.

REFERENCES

Bussey HJR, Wallace MH, Morson BC (1967). Metachronous carcinoma of the large intestine and intestinal polyps. Proc R Soc Med 60:208.

Bussey HJR (1980). Polyposis syndromes. In Wright R (ed): "Recent advances in gastrointestinal pathology," Philadelphia: WB Saunders, p 345.

Butt JH, Lennard-Jones JE, Ritchie JK (1980). A practical approach to the risk of cancer in inflammatory bowel disease. Med Clin North Am 64:1203.

Dvorak AM, Dickersin GR (1980). Crohn's disease: transmission electron microscopic studies. I. Barrier function: possible changes related to alterations of cell coat, epithelial cells and Paneth cells. Hum Pathol 11:561.

Goodman MJ, Skinner JM, Truelove SC (1976). Abnormalities in apparently normal bowel mucosa in Crohn's disease. Lancet 1:275.

Greenstein AJ, Sachar DB, Smith H, Janowtiz HD, Aufses AH Jr (1980). Patterns of neoplasia in Crohn's disease and ulcerative colitis. Cancer 46:403.

Gyde SN, Prior P, Macartney JC, Thompson H, Waterhouse JAH, Allan RN (1980). Malignancy in Crohn's disease. Gut 21:1024.

Hughes RG, Hall TJ, Block GE, Levin B, Moossa AR (1978). The prognosis of carcinoma of the colon and rectum in ulcerative colitis. Surg Gynecol Obstet 146:46.

Hulten L, Kewenter J, Ahren C (1972). Precancer and carcinoma in chronic ulcerative colitis. A histopathological and clinical investigation. Scand J Gastroenterol 7:663.

Kent TH, Mitros FA (1983). Polyps of the colon and small bowel, polyp syndromes, and the polyp-carcinoma sequence. In Norris HT (ed): "Pathology of the colon, small intestine and anus," New York:Churchill Livingstone, p 167.

Lennard-Jones JE, Ritchie JK, Morson BC, Williams CB (1983). Cancer surveillance in ulcerative colitis. Experience over 15 years. Lancet 2:149.

McManus JP (1982). Malignant problem in colitis. Gastroenterology 83:1142.

McManus JP (1984). The dilemma of dysplasia in inflammatory bowel disease. Gastroenterology 87:444.

Morson BC, Konishi F (1980). Dysplasia in the colorectum. In Wright R (ed): "Recent advances in gastrointestinal pathology," Philadelphia: WB Saunders, p 331.

Pennington L, Hamilton SR, Bayless TM, Cameron JL (1980). Surgical management of Crohn's disease: influence of disease at margin of resection. Ann Surg 192:311.

Riddell RH, Goldman H, Ransohoff DF, Appleman HD, Fenoglio CM, Haggitt RC, Ahren C, Correa P, Hamilton SR, Morson BC, Sommers SC, Yardley JH (1983). Dysplasia in inflammatory bowel disease; standardized classification with provisional clinical applciations. Hum Pathol 14:931.

Spratt JJ Jr, Ackerman LV (1962). Small primary adenocarcinoma of the colon and rectum. J Am Med Assoc 179:337.

Thayer WR Jr (1980). Malignancy in inflammatory bowel disease. In Kirsner JB, Shorter RG (eds): "Inflammatory Bowel Disease," Philadelphia: Lea and Febiger, p 265.

Weedon DD, Shorter RG, Ilstrup DM, Huizenga KA, Taylor WF (1973). Crohn's disease and cancer. N Engl J Med 289:1099.

Carcinoma of the Large Bowel and Its Precursors, pages 103–120
© 1985 Alan R. Liss, Inc.

GROWTH RATES OF BENIGN AND MALIGNANT NEOPLASMS OF THE COLON

John S. Spratt, M.D., and John A. Spratt, M.D.
J. Graham Brown Cancer Center and
Duke University Hospital

Louisville, Kentucky 40202 and
Durham, North Carolina 27710

INTRODUCTION

This study provides a review of reported data on the rates of growth of benign and malignant neoplasms of the lower bowel. These data, correlated with staging, histopathological characteristics, and prognosis are essential for understanding the extreme natural variance in the behavior of these neoplasms and for designing effective intervention programs for the control of evolving neoplasms. Data are deficient for the period elapsing between the inception of the cancer and its attainment of threshold size permitting detection. However, estimates of growth rates during this blind period can be obtained with the Gompertzian equation, and these estimates are discussed.

The sojourn time between the moment a neoplasm is large enough to detect and the moment it produces symptoms adequate to motivate a person to seek physician evaluation is known as the lead time, and the dominant determinant variable for this sojourn time is the rate of growth. Similarly, there is a critical sojourn time elapsing between the moment a neoplasm attains threshold size and the moment it disseminates beyond the region of origin and is no longer local or regional. We have designated this time as the "cancer control window" (CCW). When a virulent cancer disseminates before it reaches a threshold size permitting detection, its CCW is negative. No effective screening program would be possible for such a cancer. There is strong inferential evidence that the propensity to disseminate is inversely related to the rate of growth and is associated with histopathological characteristics. The accumulation of slow-growing neoplasms in a population contributes to length biased sampling in screening programs conducted on asymptomatic individuals. That is, the slower growing, more indolent neoplasms are the ones discovered at periodic screening. Finally, the extreme natural variance in growth rate is unequivocally associated with the extreme variance in prognosis (Spratt 1982).

To summarize the determinants of growth, a new daughter cell proceeds to a certain size and age at which binary division occurs. The process is then cyclic except that some cells die, desquamate, leave the primary mass of neoplasm via vasal or transperitoneal routes to serve as seeds for metastatic growth (Pearlman 1976; Spratt, Ackerman 1961), or become non-proliferating. Only a small percentage of cancer cells that metastasize actually survive. Cells also develop heterogeneity in their properties with successive generations. The three principal parameters determining the net rates of growth of cancer are the cell cycle time of proliferating cells, the proportion of cells proliferating, and the extent of cell loss.

The range of cell cycle time has been measured for various colonies of cancer cells. The median value (or geometric mean) of this spread is the usually quoted value. Cell cycle time is measured using tritiated thymidine to label DNA during synthesis (Steel 1972). Cytokinetic terms and their relationships are as follows:

t_c = cell cycle time.

t_s = duration of DNA synthesis of proliferating cells.

LI = the labeling index defining the ratio of the number of cells incorporating tritiated thymidine into DNA during mitosis over the total number of cells. This ratio is expressed as the percentage of cells in mitosis during the time period of thymidine incorporation.

LI = $\mu t_s/t_c$ for proliferating cells, when DT > 19 days, μ, the constant, is in the range of 0.7 to 0.8.

$DT_{(pot)}$ = potential doubling time or time required for the volume to double once in the absence of cell loss - i.e., when all dividing cells survive.

$DT_{(act)}$ = actual doubling time or actual time required for a cancer to double its volume once and represents the _net_ effect of all cytokinetic factors.

Cell loss is a major and variable factor and $DT_{(act)}$ is of longer duration thatn $DT_{(pot)}$. $DT_{(act)}$ frequently can be calculated from gross serial measurements of growing human neoplasm taken either from roentgenograms or from the direct measurement of tumor masses.

The relation between $DT_{(pot)}$ and $DT_{(act)}$ can be defined by a parameter ρ (rho) for the rate of cell loss defined as a fraction of the rate at which cells are entering mitosis. For a 100-percent loss of new cells, $DT_{(act)}$ would be static (Spratt, Spratt 1984).

The lognormal frequency distribution best describes the frequency distribution of many cytokinetic parameters as well as other characteristics of cancers and their hosts. Such a distribution occurs whenever the random errors of the variate are geometric or logarithmic rather than arithmetic or linear. These equations have been reported in detail elsewhere and their discussion is abbreviated here (Spratt, Spratt 1984).

GROWTH RATE EQUATIONS

The various growth equations express the pattern of growth within a cancer. The pattern is determined by the complex and changing interaction of variables affecting the division and accumulation of cancer cells. The number of cancer cells present, N, may be approximated by $N = 2^n$, where n is the net number of doublings of a cancer cell. When cellular replication is restricted to a peripheral margin of a growing cancer, the radius of such growth may progress at a linear rate.

Linear growth may also exist for colon cancers that grow as flat discs (cylinders). In these cancers increasing volume is primarily attributable to radial growth of a cylinder of cancer where the altitude of the cylinder (thickness of the cancer) remains relatively constant.

Cancers growing exponentially or geometrically have a steady increase in volume per unit volume per unit time. Any cell population increasing in number by the randomly steady binary division of cells, with negligible or at least steady state cell loss, would follow this equation. Spratt and Ackerman (1961) reported the first case in which the exponential growth of a primary colon cancer was confirmed.

A neoplasm following a Gompertzian (Gompertz 1925) or logistic growth grows rapidly while small but more slowly as its size increases. The curve approaches a horizontal asymptote determined by a size that the cancer never exceeds. The growth curve is upwardly concave until it reaches a point of inflection, after which it is down-wardly concave as it approaches the asymptote. In the laboratory where the kinetics of very small numbers of dividing cancer cells can be measured, Gompertzian growth is commonplace (Lloyd 1975).

Both Gompertzian and logistic curves have a sigmoid shape that characterizes many growth processes. Three adjustable parameters match growth. A close approximation of the Gompertzian or logistic curve may be obtained by matching the segments of the curve either side of the point of inflection by exponential functions. The Gompertzian growth curve follows the general equation

$$S = S_0 e^{(1-e^{-\alpha t})\beta/\alpha},$$

where S is the tumor size at time t, S_0 is the initial tumor size, and α and β are constants. The size may be expressed in any unit of measurement including number of cells. The lower asymptote is assumed to be a single cell or its volume, and the upper asymptote of the Gompertz function is obtained by letting t become artibrarily large. This theoretic limit is probably never actually attained. The constant β is the specific growth rate at $t = 0$ and approximates the clonogenic cell generation or division time. At any time t the growth rate is

$$\lambda = \beta e^{-\alpha t}$$

where λ is a proportionality factor which is dependent upon t. By differentiating the preceding general Gompert-zian equation above, the following is obtained

$$\frac{dS}{dt} = kS - \theta$$

where $k = \alpha \ln S\infty$ and $\theta = \alpha S \ln S$. In this form, k can be interpreted as an intrinsic growth rate and measures the incremental decrease in actual growth rate that occurs with increasing size. This intrinsic rate would reasonably be determined by a randomly steady rate of binary fission inherent in an asynchronously dividing clone of neoplastic cells. The actual doubling time of the neoplasm may then be determined by the following:

$$DT_{(s)} = \frac{1}{\alpha} \ln \quad (1 - \frac{\ln 2}{\ln(S\infty/S)}), \; S < 1/2 \; S^{\infty}$$

The resulting curve has a point of inflection that is rarely a concern at the gross levels of measurement. This point of inflection is attained before the cancer is gen-erally detected. Verhagen (1960) estimated the point of inflection to be at about 37 percent of the upper asymp-tote. The upper asymptote derived from clinical estimates is circa 2^{40} cells or 40 net generations. Thirty-seven percent of forty is about fifteen net generations or 2^{15} cells. Thus, the upwardly concave exponential growth period would be expected to be largely preclinical and undetectable. The segment of the growth curve measured clinically can "fit," within the random errors of limited measurement, almost any of the known possibilities.

If the point of inflection is reached at or before most cancers are grossly visible, then the exponential function applied to measurements made past the point of inflection might be sufficiently accurate for growth rate calculations, but these rates could not be used to extrapolate back and estimate time of origin of the cancer with any accuracy. However, knowing that more rapid growth may have occurred while the cancer was smaller is of great significance. A method of determining the frequency of this situation in the clinical setting is to measure the number of cancers that surface in the intervals between screening exminations, as has been done for breast cancer (Spratt et al 1982).

The Gompertzian behavior may be estimated by using various assumptions as the clonogenic rate of cellular replication ( ) at time interval elapsing between N - 2^0 and N = 2^1. This time interval (t.i.) may then be used as the unit for measuring time, t, in all equations, such that t = n(t.i.). The value of S may always be expressed as the number of cells, N = 2^n = S. The value of   can vary based on composite effects of desquamation, necrosis, cell death, and vasal dissemination of cancer cells away from the parent mass, S. The lower asymptote, S_0, approaches 2^0 and the upper asymptote, $S\infty$, exceeds a value of 2^{40} for any single contiguous colony of cancer cells in man, i.e., $2^{40} \to S\infty$.

For the value of t.i. = 1 day, the following solutions for λ may be obtained:

λ(t = 10 t.i.) = 0.83/t.i. = 1.2 days $DT_{(act)}$ when t.i. = one day. Corresponding values for t = 15, 20, or 25 t.i. are 1.64, 3.13, and 10 days $DT_{(act)}$ respectively. In this case, $DT_{(act)} = \dfrac{n(t.i.)}{\lambda}$

By time t > 30 t.i., the value of $\lambda \to 0$, and $DT_{(act)}$ correspondingly approaches infinity. Thus, with Gompertzian growth clinical cancers exceeding N = 2^{30} are slowing to the point that $DT_{(act)}$ is approaching infinity relative to the value to t.i. at inception. In fact, many colon cancers presenting as a contiguous mass of neoplastic cells are growing very slowly by the time they become radiographically measurable, and some have quit growing altogether (Welin et al 1963).

With this brief background, we may now consider available data sources and analytical observations.

METHOD

The literature was searched for reports of doubling time measurements of colonic neoplasms. The authors were surveyed to obtain the exact doubling time data which we could combine with our own for the purpose of calculating frequency distribution parameters.

Exact doubling time data were known for four of the studies (Bolin et al 1983; Burnett, Greenbaum 1981; Ekelund et al 1974, 1984; Welin et al 1963). Exact data

were not obtainable for the fifth study (Figiel 1965).
Figiel reported 18 cases but did not give summary statistics on the raw data. However, the data were displayed as
two illustrations. The doubling times are given for four
cases in one illustration. By measuring the angles
between each data point and the abscissa, the doubling
times of the remaining cases could be calculated. Of
their 18 cases, 15 are clustered into two narrow ranges
(116-118 and 404-478 days). Data from a total of 98
primary cancers were obtained for study.

The literature was also surveyed in order to obtain
doubling time data on pulmonary metastases from colonic
adenocarcinomas. Exact data were obtained for 23 cases
from a total of six studies (Brenner 1971; Breur 1966;
Chahinian 1982; Collins 1962; Joseph 1971; Spratt, Spratt
1964). In addition, actual doubling time data were known
for 77 colonic polyps from one study (Welin et al, 1963).
These polyps were mostly adenomatous polyps but included
seven villous adenomas as well. Data from a total of 98
adenomas were obtained.

Once the doubling time for the pooled data in each of
three histological groups was obtained, the statistical
analyses were performed. The first was to calculate the
mean, standard deviation, and range for the doubling times
and the logarithms of the doubling times. Summary data
are shown in Table 1. The arithmetic mean of the doubling
times is expressed in days. The geometric mean is the
exponential of the mean of the logarithm of the doubling
times. The geometric mean is a better measure of central
tendency in this setting.

TABLE 1

	Geomet-ric Mean (days)	Mean In (D.T.)	S.D. In (D.T.)	Maxi-mum (days)	Mini-mum (days)	Arith-metic Mean (days)	n
Cancer	352	5.92	0.99	10000	52	668	98
Polyps	946	6.85	1.13	8664	13	1600	77
Metas-tases	85	4.45	0.93	3300	32	221	23

Histograms of the raw data for each histological type
are shown in Figure 1. The cumulative probability

distributions of the logarithm of the same data were determined. The next step performed was to test each group for a significant difference from the normal distribution. This was done using the Kolmogarov-Smirnov test. Summary statistics are shown in Table 2. Tests for skewness and kurtosis were also performed.

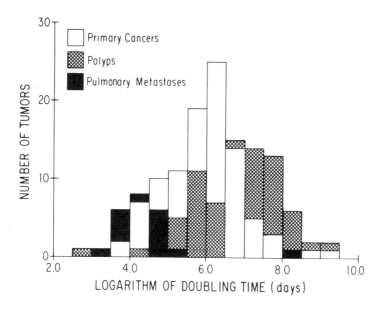

Fig. 1. Histogram of logarithm of doubling time in days for primary cancers, polyps, and pulmonary metastases.

TABLE 2

	D_{Max}	P	Skewness	P	Kurtosis	P
Cancer	0.0681	>0.20	0.401	0.100	0.777	0.108
Polyps	0.0743	>0.20	-0.688	0.012	1.746	0.000
Metastases	0.2231	0.01	2.910	0.001	11.160	0.000

In the final portion of the analysis, the means of each group were tested with the Kruskal-Wallace test. Differences in the distributions were tested with the two-sample Kolmogorov-Smirnov test. The type-I error rate was controlled with Bonferroni's inequality.

RESULTS

In Table 1, the geometric mean doubling time for colonic cancers was 372 days, while it was much slower for adenomas and much faster for pulmonary metastases. Differences between these means were statistically significant (P < 0.05) in all instances. The statistical analysis used to make these comparisons does not require a known distribution function for the data so that no assumptions of a normal distribution have been made. The differences in means of the logarithm of doubling times can also be appreciated from Figure 1. The pulmonary metastases data are clustered to the left, with a peak incidence of four to five. The primary cancers have a peak incidence at approximately six, and the polyps are just to the right at approximately seven.

The cumulative probability density distributions were next analyzed and each was seen to be statistically significantly different from the others (P < 0.05). This allows us to say that the distribution of doubling times of colonic neoplasms are different depending upon histology. Pulmonary metastases grow most quickly, followed by primary cancers, then colonic polyps.

The final portion of the analysis tested each of the cumulative probability density functions for normality. These data are shown in Table 2. As can be seen, the cancer data are not statistically significantly different from normal (P > 0.20). Tests for skewness and kurtosis were also not significant. This test has an approximate power of 0.7 to detect a difference from normality with $\alpha = 0.05$. We may therefore state that the lognormal distribution is a close approximation to the naturally occurring distribution of the actual doubling times of colonic cancers that have achieved a size large enough to measure by double contrast enema. A similar analysis for the adenoma data again showed no significant difference from the lognormal (P > 0.20), but the power of this test is not as great due to the smaller sample size. The polyp data also showed significant skewness and kurtosis. The same tests were applied for pulmonary metastases showing a significant difference from normality existed (P < 0.01). This is due largely to the fact that one doubling time measurement was 3000 days, which is far greater than the others.

RATES OF GROWTH OF PRIMARY CANCERS

Many small, well-differentiated adenocarcinomas of the colon grow predominantly as plaques. While small, the plaques may wrinkle over their submucosal stroma and some may even develop pedicles, making them grossly indistinguishable from pedunculated benign adenomatous polyps (Spratt, Ackerman 1960a). Later the central part of the plaque desquamates while the cancer grows beneath and around the erosion, with a tendency toward circumferential spread. The volume of such a cancer can be calculated from the roentgen films after correcting for magnification simply by treating the lesion as a cylinder having a diameter (d) ascertained from the roentgenogram and a depth (h) equal to the thickness of the tumor measured after its removal (Spratt, Ackerman 1961).

In the Malmö data (Welin, et al 1963), the greatest tumor diameter and the dates of measurements on two or more double contrast enema studies were recorded for 136 colonic tumors excised from 109 patients. For 239 untreated tumors in 194 patients, measurements were also made.

The time intervals between examinations were recorded in days. At Malmö, semiannual reexamination of patients with tumors was encouraged, but this policy was not followed strictly. The number of double contrast enema studies for each patient varied from two (215 patients) to 10 (one patient). Only 10 tumors were observed for a total period of less than 6 months.

Since the distribution function for the cancer data is known with some accuracy, the mean doubling time and 95 percent confidence intervals of the mean can be estimated. These data are shown in Figure 1 and the probability distribution has been determined and is separately available. The mean doubling time is 372 days and the 95 percent confidence interval estimates of the mean are 51 days and 2,711 days. This indicates that 95 percent of all colonic cancers will have a doubling time within this range by the time they are grossly measurable by double contrast enema. This range is obviously very large and should be kept in mind when studying clinical series advocating efficacy of a particular treatment for colonic cancers. Due to the large natural variability, a significant proportion of patients could be expected to do well in the absence of any treatment.

RATES OF GROWTH OF PULMONARY METASTASES

As early as 1956, Collins, et al reported the time required for a pulmonary metastases from four rectal adenocarcinomas to double in volume. The time ranged from 49 to 123 days. In 1962, Collins updated his investigations and by that time had 25 cases of rectal cancer. The doubling times ranged from 34 to 210 days with a median of 96 days.

In the present study, doubling times of pulmonary metastases ranged from 32-3300 days, with mean of log-normal frequency distribution of doubling times of 85 days.

Collins, et al (1956) speculated on time of origin of pulmonary metastases by extrapolating backwards with his doubling time data. They took the doubling times of the pulmonary metastases and made the assumption that, if the doubling time remained constant from the moment of metastasis and if the original size of a metastasis was a single cell, the time of occurrence of the metastasis could be estimated. By his estimates, pulmonary metastases could have occurred from 3 to 18 years before discovery of the primary cancer. He considered this a fundamental reason why mortality rates were not changing despite other advances in the period. He observed that the prescriptions for earlier and more radical surgery and earlier detection as means of lowering mortality rates should "offer some assurance that the techniques and tools at hand are equal to the demand placed upon them" (Collins 1962). Although this conclusion may be correct, his extrapolations of duration were too long because he did not consider Gompertzian growth. A more definitive way of estimating duration before diagnosis is to divide the prevalence rate by the annual incidence rate assuming that the incidence rate remains constant (Spratt 1982; Spratt, Ackerman 1962; Spratt, Spratt 1984). This value has been estimated to range from 6.8 to 65 years for primary colonic cancers (Spratt 1982).

As mentioned earlier, the basic assumption that exponential growth is constant from the inception of the neoplasm is false. The extremely early phase of cancer may proceed at a much faster rate. The rate then slows with increasing size and as the tumor becomes grossly measurable.

DISCUSSION

The collected data defined changes in diameter over measured periods of time. The authors recognized that they were measuring the net results of new cell formation (the fundamental requisite for growth), cell death, cell dissemination away from the primary, and surface desquamation. Generally, when cellular proliferation is unrestrained growth proceeds by geometric progression, or exponential increase in the numbers of cells, and the rate of increase is constantly proportional to the size already attained. When growth limiting factors slow the growth of increasingly large neoplasms, Gompertzian or logistic growth occurs. Other variables acting simultaneously could alter the exponential growth to produce any of the variety of types of growth mentioned previously including arithmetic or linear growth in the diameter, random variation in growth, continued deceleration in growth, continued acceleration in growth, Gompertzian growth, or no growth (Davis 1960; Defares, Sneddon 1960; Gompertz 1825; Hoffman 1953; Mayneord 1932; Spratt, Spratt 1964; Verhagen 1960). The ability to determine the growth curves best fitting the collected data is hampered by the limited number of measurements and the absence of in vivo data on growth in the period preceding gross visibility.

First, the geometric configuration of growing colonic neoplasms has to be known to relate the chordal dimensions to changes in tumor volume. Most cancers of the colon and rectum grow over the mucosal surface of bowel as circumferentially spreading plaques. The plaques become ulcerated, sessile or pedunculated (Spratt, Ackerman 1962). The plaques approached the geometric shape of cylinders ("medallion cancers") until they achieved a diameter of several centimeters. At this size, some of them were prone to involve the entire circumference of the bowel ("napkin ring" cancers). These surface-spreading growths remained fairly constant in thickness, and the changing volumes of the growing cancers were mainly proportional to the surface areas. In analyzing these Malmö data, the authors regarded the diameters measured as being the diameters of the bases of cylinders of uniform thickness. More simply, they regarded change in surface area as being directly proportional to change in volume in cancers of constant thickness.

A concern with these data is that nothing is known about the rate of growth of tumors seen only once on a barium enema before removal. If these were faster growing neoplasms, then frequency distributions of growth rates would be truncated. Also, not known are the number of cancers that surfaced in the intervals between barium enemas and produced symptoms leading to discovery and resection. These interval-surfacing cancers could grow even faster than the previously mentioned tumors. They might well come to emergency operations with no roentgen measurements at all.

Obviously, many elderly people would be expected to die with, although not from, these indolent slow-growing neoplasms in their colon and rectum. That this occurs is confirmed by the high prevalence of asymptomatic colonic neoplasms found at the autopsy of elderly people but never diagnosed in the antemortem state.

The vast majority of the benign adenomatous polyps grow so slowly that they could not have achieved a significant size during the longest human life span. This indolent or slow growth would also permit significant accumulation of asymptomatic benign adenomas in the aging colon producing the very high prevalence rates found when the colons of the elderly are screened using double contrast enemas, flexible endoscopes or are examined by autopsy. These very indolent tumors often produce and desquamate new glandular cells without increasing in mass. To this extent they behave as normal intestinal epithelium. However, sometime in the life history of these tumors, they had to enlarge enough to become visible.

Failure of slowly growing or non-growing noninvasive tumors to attain significant size during the human life span has practical significance in the diagnosis of colonic tumors demonstrated by double contrast enema studies or endoscopic observation. Very slow growing tumors do not get very big. The measurement of fresh tissue specimens of consecutively resected benign and malignant tumors showed that benign tumors exceeded a diamenter of 12 mm infrequently (Spratt, Ackerman 1960b). With an error in roentgenographic measurement of ±2 mm, the critical dimension should lie in the vicinity of 10-14 mm. An analysis of the diameters of the 375 tumors in the Malmo study measured on the first and the last of the serial double contrast enema studies showed the critical roentgenographic diameter to be 10 mm. Tumors larger than 10 mm were undergoing sustained growth, and there was a greater chance of their being invasive cancers. One of the two cancers that was 10 mm or less in diameter developed marginal infiltration before it attained a diameter of 10 mm, permitting the diagnosis of cancer based on roentgenographic appearance.

As previously observed, the diagnosis of cancer has been made correctly on the basis of infiltrating margins seen on double contrast enemas in tumors as small as 3 mm in diameter. However, pedunculated cancers, cancers with well-circumscribed or pushing margins, and cancers arising in villous adenomas may not develop this sign until they are quite large. In these cases, when biopsy is not possible, we must rely on size and growth to make the diagnosis of cancer. The statistical chance that any polypoid tumor attaining a roentgenographic diameter greater than 10 mm is a cancer is so great that resection is indicated on the basis of size alone. Search for other roentgenographic evidence of cancer would be superfluous. Tumors smaller than 10 mm in diameter and appearing benign roentgenographically may be observed safely by serial double contrast enema studies. Many will disappear spontaneously (Welin, et al 1963). Only those that grow with a cancerous rate of growth or that exceed a diameter of 10 mm on subsequent examinations will require resection. Among the numerous very small tumors (less than 8 mm in diameter) with no premalignant significance, (Koppel, et al 1962; Spratt, et al 1958) new cancers have been found with the same age-specific incidence rates observed for the general population (Spratt, Ackerman 1962). However, in children, single and multiple retention polyps regularly exceed a diameter of 10 mm. Roentgenographically, these tumors appear benign. They have been observed until disappearance (Welin 1958).

Transendoscopic removal of all tumors, no matter how small, for histopathologic evaluation is possible, as long as they are visible by endoscope. No controlled clinical trial for screening intervention was defined as the optimum strategy for reducing the mortality from colonic cancer. The frequency of small, non-growing, benign colonic tumors is so great that no morbidity or mortality as a result of their removal as a means of cancer prevention is justified. If it occurs, the value of the screening effort may be negative.

Computerized Axial Tomography (CAT) Scans

Sequential computerized tomography has provided still another means of generating growth rate data. Havelaar, et al (1984) monitored the progression and regression of intra-abdominal metastases from colorectal cancer in four patients. The $DT_{(act)}$ for untreated patients varied from 50 to 95 days. They also established the feasibility monitoring regression that paralleled the fall in CEA in response to FUDR. They suggested that failure to demonstrate regression would merit discontinuance of the therapy in progress.

SUMMARY

In summary, there is a wide, natural variance in rates of growth of benign and malignant neoplasms of the lower bowel. There is a crude correlation between growth rate and histopathology. The difference between $DT_{(act)}$ and $DT_{(pot)}$ is manifold. Primary surface desquamating cancers probably grow much slower than their metastases. These factors are of importance in understanding neoplastic behavior and in designing detection and treatment protocols. The gap in knowledge is for in vivo growth rates and mathematical patterns of growth in the period before a neoplasm reaches the threshold size permitting observation. The rates of growth are very relevant to screening and diagnostic strategies.

REFERENCES

Bolin S, Nilsson E, Sjodahl R (1983). Carcinoma of the colon and rectum-growth rate. Ann Surg 198:151158.

Brenner MW, Holsti LR, Perttala Y (1971). Variation in tumor doubling time in patients with pulmonary metastatic disease. J Surg Oncol 3:143-149.

Breur K (1966). Growth rate and radiosensitivity of human tumours--I. Eur J Cancer Clin Oncol 2:157-171.

Burnett KR, Greenbaum EI (1981). Rapidly growing carcinoma of the colon. Dis Colon Rectum 24:282-286.

Chahinian P (1982). Relationship between tumor doubling time and anatomoclinical features in 50 measurable pulmonary cancers. Chest 51:340-345.

Collins VP (1962). Time of occurrence of pulmonary metastases from carcinoma of colon and rectum. Cancer 15:387-395.

Collins VP, Loeffler RK, Tivey H (1956). Observations on growth rates of human tumors. AJR 76:988-1000.

Davis HT (1960). Problem of growth in two populations conflicting with one another. In "Introduction of Nonlinear Differential and Integral Equations," Washington, D.C.: U.S. Government Printing Office, p. 99-102.

Defares JG, Sneddon IN (1960). Common growth and biology. In "An Introduction to the Mathematics of Medicine and Biology," Chicago: Yearbook Publishers, p. 227-234.

Ekelund G, Lindstrom C, Rosengren JE (1974). Appearance and growth of early carcinomas of the colon-rectum. Acta Radiol (Diagn) 15:670-679, and personal communication.

Figiel LS, Figiel SJ, Wietersen FK (1965). Roentgenologic observations of growth rates of colonic polyps and carcinoma. Acta Radiol [Diagn] 3:417-429.

Gompertz B (1825). On the nature of the function expressive of the law of human mortality, and on a new method of determining the value of life contingencies. Philos Trans R Soc Lond 513-585.

Havelaar IJ, Sugarbaker PH, Vermess J, and Miller DL (1984). Rate of growth of intraabdominal metastases from colorectal cancer. Cancer 54:163-171.

Hoffman JG (1949). Theory of the mitotic index and its application to tissue growth measurement. Bull Math Biol 11:139-144.

Joseph WL, Morton DL, Adkins PC (1971). Variation in tumor doubling time in patients with pulmonary metastatic disease. J Surg Oncol 3:143-149.

Koppel M, Bailar JC III, Weakley FL, Shimkin MB (1962). Incidence of cancer in colon and rectum among polyp-free patients. Dis Colon Rectum 5:349-355.

Lloyd HH (1975). Estimation of tumor cell kill from Gompertz growth curves. Cancer Chemother Rep 59(2 Pt 1), 267-277.

Mayneord WV (1932). On a law of growth of Jensen's rat sarcoma. Am J Cancer 16:841-846.

Pearlman AW (1976). Breast cancer--influence of growth rate on prognosis and treatment evaluation. A study based on mastectomy scar recurrences. Cancer 38:1826-1833.

Ravikumar T, Steele G, Rodrick M, Ross D, Wilson R, Lahey S, Wright D, Munroe A, and King V (1984). Effects of tumor growth on interleukins and circulating immune complexes--mechanisms of immune unresponsiveness. Cancer 53:1373-1378.

Spratt JS (1982). Epidemiology of screening for cancer. Curr Probl Cancer 6:1-58.

Spratt JS Jr, Ackerman LV (1960a). Pathological significance of polyps of the rectum and colon. Dis Colon Rectum 3:330-335.

Spratt JS Jr, Ackerman LV (1960b). Relationship of size of colonic tumors to their cellular composition and biological behavior. Surg Forum 10:56-61.

Spratt JS Jr, Ackerman LV (1961). The growth of a colonic adenocarcinoma. Am Surg 27:23-28.

Spratt JS JR, Ackerman LV (1962). Small primary adenocarcinomas of colon and rectum. JAMA 179:337-346.

Spratt JS JR, Ackerman LV, Moyer CA (1958). Relationship of polyps of colon to colonic cancers. Ann Surg 148:682-698.

Spratt JS, Heuser L, Kuhns JG, Greenberg R, Polk HC Jr, Buchanan JB (1982). Variations and associations in histopathology clinical factors, mammographic patterns and growth rates among breast cancers confirmed in a screened population. In "Issues in Cancer Screening Communications," New York: Alan R. Liss, pp. 295-299.

Spratt JS JR, Spratt JA (1984). Growth rates. In Spratt JS Jr, "Neoplasms of the colon, rectum and anus," Philadelphia: W. B. Saunders Co., pp. 24-44.

Spratt JS JR, Spratt TL (1964). Rates of growth of pulmonary metastases and host survival. Ann Surg 159:161-171.

Steel GG (1972). The cell cycle in tumours: an examination of data gained by the technique of labeled mitosis. Cell Tissue Kinet 5:87-100.

Taylor CW, Brittain MG, Yeoman LC (1984). Rate of growth and extent of differentiation reflected by cytoplasmic proteins, and antigens of human colon tumor cell lines. Cancer Res 44:1200-1205.

Verhagen AMV (1960). Growth curves and their functional forms. Aust J Stat 2:122-127.

Welin S (1958). Modern trends in diagnostic roentgenology of colon. The Mackenzie Davidson Memorial Lecture. Br J Radiol 31:453-464.

Welin S, Youker J, Spratt JS Jr, Linell F, Spjut HJ, Johnson RE, Ackerman LV (1963). The rates and patterns of growth of 375 tumors of the large intestine and rectum observed serially by double contrast enema study (Malmo Technique). AJR 90:673-687.

Carcinoma of the Large Bowel and Its Precursors, pages 121–132
© **1985 Alan R. Liss, Inc.**

COLONOSCOPY: ITS APPLICATION AND MERIT

John Stroehlein, M.D.
Asst. Professor of Medicine
Baylor College of Medicine
Director Digestive Disease Laboratory
  and Endoscopy Unit, The Methodist Hospital
Houston Texas 77030

INTRODUCTION

The application and merits of colonoscopy are still being assessed: however, since this procedure was intro- duced approximately sixteen years ago it has proven to be very valuable clinically and informative about the devel- opment of colorectal neoplasia.

Application and merit of colonoscopy will be discuss- ed from the standpoint of several situations including its use in patients with unexplained rectal bleeding, cancer, adenoma(s) at high risk of cancer, and as an investiga- tional tool.

CLINICAL AND INVESTIGATIONAL USE

A. Occult or Overt Lower GI Bleeding:

Application: For patients with acute colonic bleeding whose bleeding does not significantly obscure the visual field or those with intermittent bleeding colonoscopy is often applied in an effort to determine the cause of bleeding if the cause is not obvious by unprepared proctoscopy. Colonoscopy is often preferred in this setting because it permits performing angiography without additional preparation. As will be discussed, neoplasms are the most common cause of colonic bleeding and can be histologically diagnosed by colonoscopic biopsies. Poly- pectomy and electro or photocoagulation of benign or malignant lesions represent therapeutic applications of colonoscopy performed for colonic bleeding.

Merit: The merits of colonoscopy in determining the cause of colonic bleeding are based on diagnostic yield, frequency of neoplasia as a cause of colonic bleeding, and therapeutic potential of the procedure. In three large series of over 200 patients each (Tedesco 1978; Hunt 1980; Brand 1980) colonoscopy identified the presence of carcinoma in about 10% of individuals with negative barium examination performed for colonic bleeding. Similar merit has been described for occult bleeding in the over 50 age group (Winawer 1980, Stroehlein 1984). Almost one-third of colonic neoplasms causing hematochezia are proximal to the sigmoid (Tedesco 1980). Consequently, examination of the entire colon is advised if the cause of hematochezia is not clearly established by sigmoidoscopy. The significance of neoplasia as a common cause of colonic bleeding is discussed below: the therapeutic role of colonscopy will be discussed elsewhere in this book.

Perspective: The colonoscopic identification of pathology not apparent on barium contrast examination in patients with rectal bleeding should come as no surprise. Similarly a negative colonoscopy for patients who have rectal bleeding does not always exclude the presence of pathology which may be identified by barium contrast examination. This is related to the fact that prevalence or probability of disease in a patient population influences the positive and negative predictive value of the diagnostic test being performed. In other words, if a disease is more likely to be present, this influences the predictive value of a test - be it colonoscopy or barium contrast examination.

This is illustrated by a hypothetical example using a test with 80% sensitivity and 80% specificity wherein one can see, by comparing the following two examples, how the probable presence or absence of a condition affects the predictive value when the sensitivity and specificity are unchanged.

Example 1: Very unlikely (1:9) that a
condition is present using a test with
sensitivity 80% and specificity 80%.

	Condition		
	Present 100	Absent 900	Predictive Value (PV)
Test Pos	80	180	31% (Pos.PV)
Test Neg	20	720	97% (Neg.PV)

Example 2: Even chances (50:50) that a
condition is present using a test with the
same, i.e., 80% sensitivity and specificity.

	Condition		
	Present 500	Absent 500	Predictive Value
Test Pos	400	100	80% (Pos PV)
Test Neg	100	400	80% (Neg PV)

These examples illustrate the fact that an unexpect-
edly negative study is more likely to be a false negative
With respect to colonic bleeding, about one-fourth of
patients with chronic intermittent or acute colonic
bleeding have neoplasia (Tedesco 1978; Forde 1981) and
occult bleeding in the over 50 age group is most commonly
a manifestation of colonic bleeding and this most commonly
due to neoplasia (Stroehlein 1984). Several studies have
demonstrated the advantage of total colonoscopy when a
barium enema is non-diagnostic or reveals only diverticula
(Teague 1978; Tedesco 1978; Brand 1980). A more recent
prospective study has confirmed that colonoscopy is more
sensitive than barium enema and can be effectively
utilized as the initial study in patients with nonactive
lower intestinal bleeding (Tedesco 1984). Barium contrast
examination may be critical in achieving visualization of
the entire colon when full colonoscopy cannot be performed
and when done carefully barium examination achieves a high
accuracy at limited cost.

B. Colorectal Cancer

Application: Colonoscopy with biopsy and/or poly-

pectomy is applied to histologically confirm the presence
of malignancy, identify the more than 1 in 50 cancer patients who will have a synchronous cancer (Moertel 1958)
and more than 1 in 2 who will have at least one associated
adenoma (Reilly 1982). Following surgery for cancer,
anastomotic recurrence is unusual if adequate cancer free
margins were resected: however, metachronous lesions occur
in at least 2% of cases and, in time, as many as 5 or 10%.

Merit: Colonsocopy has the merit of establishing a
tissue diagnosis and removing adenomas that would not
otherwise be in the operative field. This saves operative
time and helps establish the extent of surgery. The
examination also has the merit of being performed in conjunction with a single preoperative bowel preparation. In
selected cases of rectal cancer therapeutic endoscopy may
be palliative or curative when performed in conjunction
with radiotherapy (Papillon J 1980).

Perspective: Preoperatively establishing a diagnosis
of cancer permits cancer surgery to be more effectively
planned and performed. Definitive preoperative diagnosis
may not improve survival which is dependent on the stage
of disease at diagnosis: however, it facilitates and
defines the extent of surgery. Postoperative colonoscopy
provides the ability to remove adenomas and offers the
best chance for cure of metachronous cancers which must be
identified before symptoms develop in order to maximize
the possibility of cure. Metachronous cancers are no
different than an initial cancer with respect to the
importance of establishing a diagnosis before symptoms
develop. Over three-fourths of patients whose cancers are
discovered while asymptomatic will have early Dukes' A or
B lesions and an overall 5-year survival approaching 70-
80% (Copeland EM III 1968: Murray D 1975). Because of the
high risk of metachronous lesions in patients who have
undergone resection for colon cancer, surveillance must
include periodic visualization of the remaining portion of
the colon by barium enema or colonoscopy.

C. Adenomas

Application: Size is a reasonably good indicator of
benignancy of colorectal polyps but it is not the reliable
indicator of histology it was once considered to be (Wayne

1980; Brady; 1980). In addition, the distribution of adenomas (as opposed to hyperplastic polyps) is fairly even throughout the large bowel and there is a 40% chance of synchronous lesions when an index adenoma is found (Miller 1980; Waye 1980; Williams AR 1982).

Once cleared of all polyps about one-third of patients will develop new lesions. These observations have lead to the practice of removing all polyps exceeding 5mm and placing the patient on long-term surveillance.

Merit; Although not error free, colonoscopy is generally about 12% more accurate than barium enema from a false negative plus a false positive standpoint in identifying lesions under 1 cm (Williams 1974; Hogan 1977; Theoni 1977). An important prospective study of diagnostic methods in 330 adenoma follow-up patients at St. Mark's Hospital involved concurrent air contrast barium enema colonoscopy. Of 63 lesions greater than 7mm, 5 were missed by colonoscopy and 17 by barium enema (Williams CB 1982). Accuracy notwithstanding, the merit of colonoscopy rests on the therapeutic implications of polypectomy.

Perspective: Colonoscopy and air contrast barium examination are very operator dependent. This makes it difficult to compare studies; however, for the established adenoma patient colonoscopy has certain advantages which include increased yield and therapeutic potential. The relative importance of removing all small adenomas and frequency of follow-up have yet to be firmly established; however, evidence indicates that most carcinomas develop from adenomas - a process which appears to invariably require years (Kozuka 1975). Removing these neoplastic potentially premalignant lesions is anticipated to reduce the incidence of invasive cancer (Gilbertsen 1974; Kronborg 1980). Prospective data regarding the impact of colonoscopic polypectomy for prophylaxis of colorectal cancer are lacking. Only a small percentage of adenomas become cancers and it is now apparent that some patients are at greater risk than others. Stratification of follow-up for high and low risk individuals has been developed (Lambert 1984). Those at high risk include patients with any of the following: Multiple adenomas at initial polypectomy; adenoma equal or greater than two cm; sessile lesions; presence of dysplasia; carcinoma in situ or invasive cancer in an adenoma. It is anticipated that

colonoscopic polypectomy will have an impact on the incidence of colon cancer and that optimal follow-up programs
can be more precisely established for individual patients.

D. Inflammatory Bowel Disease

Application: Treatment and surveillance of idiopathic
inflammatory bowel disease is highly dependent on making an
accurate diagnosis and establishing the extent of disease.
Colonoscopy can be effectively applied to these situations
because it provides visualization of gross pathology and
procurement of tissue. Histopathological interpretation
may be diagnostic of a specific type of colitis or help to
differentiate Crohn's disease from CUC when idiopathic
colitis is present (Haggitt 1983). Furthermore abnormalities such as changes in crypt architecture may be the
only sign of previous involvement. This can be very
important in establishing extent of disease and making
decisions regarding surveillance.

Variations in incidence notwithstanding, it is uniformly accepted that patients who have CUC are at increased risk of developing cancer (Devroede 1971; Riddell
1976; Katzka 1983). The overall occurrence is about 4%
(Goldgraber 1964; Riddell 1983). Even in the highest risk
subgroup, where the risk increases about twenty percent/
decade, only a minority will develop cancer. This cannot
be predicted by clinical parameters. Because precursor
lesions are often associated with cancer, it was initially
suggested in 1949 that precursor lesions antedate the
development of cancer in CUC (Warren 1949). In 1967, the
precancerous changes of CUC were accurately described
(Morson 1967). Subsequent retrospective and prospective
studies have revealed (a) about a 35% incidence of unsuspected cancer in patients with dysplasia on rectal biopsy;
(b) the importance of plaque or mass lesions (Blackstone
1981); and (c) the nonuniform distribution of dysplasia
(Riddell 1983; Blackstone 1981). Because of the lack of
clinical criteria in determining individual risk and the
strong association of premalignant changes and cancer
complicating CUC, colonoscopy is periodically applied to
detect precancerous changes before invasive malignancy.

Merit: One merit of colonoscopy is the ability to
sample all portions of the colon. As indicated above,

dysplastic changes are not uniform and have been identified more than three times as often at colonoscopy as opposed to just rectal biopsy (Hanauer 1984). Plaque or mass-like lesions - be they identified at colonoscopy or barium enema - carry an increased probability of associated cancer or dysplasia and require biopsy. Mild dysplasia associated with a gross lesion has significance similar to moderately severe dysplasia. Colonoscopy has the merit of obtaining directed biopsies of these mass or plaque-like lesions. Colonoscopy can also resolve the nature of strictures - submucosal cancer notwithstanding - and other abnormalities encountered on barium enema because of the ability to obtain tissue. Encoscopic polypectomy for adenoma(s) complicating CUC provides the opportunity to perform macroscopic biopsy which should be combined with biopsies of the surrounding mucosa to determine if the adenoma associated with CUC is secondary to dysplasia or not. The merit of colonoscopy involves the fact that tissue confirmation is essential in the diagnosis of idiopathic inflammatory bowel disease determining the extent of disease and conducting surveillance for dysplasia.

Perspective: The impact of colonoscopy with multiple biopsies on survival in patients who have inflammatory bowel disease is yet to be established. The experience to date indicates that this is clinically useful - particularly for patients who are at increased risk for cancer but have relatively quiescent disease and no additional indications for surgery. When the colon is removed for dysplasia, the stage of unsuspected cancer in two-thirds of the cases has been reported to be Dukes' A or B (Fuson 1980). Although there is considerable merit in sampling all segments of the colon endoscopically, colonoscopy as opposed to sigmoidoscopy has not been prospectively established to enhance survival. Pending more definitive data and establishing survival, cost-benefit and cost-analysis ratios, colonoscopy with multiple biopsies in CUC patients is considered (a) superior to prophylactic colectomy or simple observation, and (b) indicated when a definitive diagnosis has yet to be established - lest therapy for a specific type of colitis be neglected or steroid therapy be responsible for accentuating an infectious process. When a diagnosis cannot be established by sigmoidoscopy and barium contrast examination, colonoscopy can typically resolve the dilemma and establish extent of disease.

E. Proliferative Abnormality:

Application: Cellular proliferation patterns and chromosomal abnormalities can serve as biologically indicators of neoplasia, precancerous conditions and changes induced by investigational intervention. Mucosal biopsies obtained during endoscopy are adequate for assessing nuclear ploidy using flow cytometry (Bennetts 1979), changes in proliferative activity, which accompany adenoma formation and inflammatory bowel disease (Deschner 1980; Deschner 1983; Sherlock 1980), assay for ornithine decarboxylase (Luk 1984), chromosomal changes associated with neopolasia (Reichmann 1980) and determination of human colonic mucin glycoprotein heterogeneity (Podolsky 1984).

Merit: Studying the evolution of large bowel cancer provides a better understanding of preneoplastic proliferative abnormalities and factors which influence their development. Intervention designed to affect these changes can also be examined using colonoscopy since it permits procurement of tissue for sequential observations in large animal models and clinical studies using patients as their own controls.

Perspective: Historically many potential markers of early cancer or cancer risk have been studied and eventually not been found to be of value. Many of these studies antedated our ability to sequentially sample the colonic epithelial target tissue from grossly normal and abnormal tissue in all portions of the colon. This is now possible. With advanced technique and this ability, it is possible that kinetic parameters may eventually supplement histopathology in assessing risk for future neoplasia or modifying the proliferative activity of the normal colon and the cell cycle of cancer. In the future, it may also be possible to examine (a) the effect of trophic agents, including gastrointestinal hormones which are known to have a trophic effect on normal colonic mucosa (Johnson 1978) and malignant (McGregor 1982) colonic epithelium; (b) inhibitors of critical enzyme systems (Luk 1984); or (c) determinations of mucin profiles which may be characteristically altered in certain colonic disorders (Podolsky 1984).

SUMMARY

Much has been learned through the development of colonoscopy. This in turn has stimulated interest in roentgenographic studies and has provided a tool for conducting research studies that would not be possible without the ability to obtain tissue sequentially over a period of time. Despite these advances, questions still outnumber answers. As new technologies open doors for research that was not historically possible, commitment to research in endoscopy becomes increasingly important. The opportunities, importance and need for commitment to endoscopic research has recently been emphasized (Silverstein 1984). It is hoped that important research questions in endoscopy will be effectively addressed and this, in turn, will improve our knowledge about cancer of the large bowel and its precursors.

REFERENCES

Bennetts RW, Stroehlein J, Barlogie B (1979). Ploidy determination by DNA flow cytometry of malignant and benign gastric tissue obtained by endoscopic biopsy. Gastroenterol 76:1099.

Blackstone MO, Riddell RH, Rogers BHG et al (1981). Dysplasia-associated lesion or mass (DALM) detected by colonoscopy in long-standing ulcerative colitis: An indication for colectomy. Gastroenterol 80:366-374.

Brady PG (1980). The significance of minute colonic polyps. Gastrointest Endosc 26:64.

Brand EJ, Sullivan BH, Sivak MV, Rankin GB (1980) Colonoscopy in the diagnosis of unexplained rectal bleeding. Ann Surg 192:111-113.

Copeland EM III, Miller LD, Jones RS (1968). Prognostic factors in carcinoma of the colon and rectum. Amer J of Surg 116:865-881.

Deschner EE (1980). Cell proliferation as a biological marker in human colorectal neoplasia. In Winawer SJ, Schottenfeld P, Sherlock P (eds): "Colorectal Cancer: Prevention, Epidemiology and Screening", Raven Press, New York pp 133-142.

Deschner EE (1983). Adenomas. Preneoplastic events, growth characteristics, and development. Pathol Annual 13:205-219.

Devroede GJ, Taylor WF, Sauer WG et al (1971) Cancer risk and life expectancy of children with ulcerative colitis. N Engl J Med 285:17-21

Forde KA (1981). Colonoscopy in acute rectal bleeding. Gastrointest Endosc 27:219-220.

Fuson JA, Farmer RG, Sullivan BH (1980). Endoscopic surveillance for cancer in chronic ulcerative colitis Amer J Gastro 73:120-126.

Gilbertsen VA (1974) Proctosigmoidoscopy and polypectomy in reducing invasive rectal cancer. Cancer 34:936-939.

Goldgraber MB, Kirsner JB (1964). Carcinoma of the colon in ulcerative colitis. Cancer 17:657-665.

Haggitt RC (1983). The differential diagnosis of idiopathic inflammatory bowel disease in pathology of colon, small intestine and anus. In Norris HT (ed): "Churchill Livingstone", New York, NY pp 21-59.

Hanauer SB, Levin B, Evans AA, Riddell RH, Kirsner JB (1984). Location of dysplasia at colonoscopy compared to surgical resection: inadequacy of rectal biopsy to predict proximal lesions. Gastroenterol 86(5):1106.

Hogan WJ, Stewart ET, Geenew JE, Dodds WJ, Biork JT, Leinicke JA (1977). A prospective comparison of the accuracy of colonoscopy vs. air-barium contrat exam for detection of colonic polypoid lesions. Gastrointest Endosc 23:230

Hunt RH, Swarbrick ET, Teague RH, Thomas BM. Thornton JR, Williams CB (1980). Colonoscopy for unexplained rectal bleeding. Gastroenterol 76:1158.

Johnson LR, Copeland EM, Dudrick SJ (1978). Luminal gastrin stimulates growth of distal rat intestine. Scand J Gastroenterol (Supple 49)13:95.

Katzka I, Brody RS, Katz S (1983). An assessment of colorectal cancer in patients with ulcerative colitis: experience from a private practice. Gastroenterol 85:22-29.

Kozuka S, Nogaki M, Ozeki T et al (1975). Premalignancy of the mucosal polyp in the large intestine. II. Estimation of the periods required for malignant transformation of mucosal polyps. Dis Colon Rectum 18:494-500.

Kronborg O (1980). Polyps of the colon and rectum: approach to prophylaxis in colorectal cancer. Scand J Gastroenterol 15:1-5.

Lambert R, Sobin LH, Waye JD, Stalder GA (1984). The management of patients with colorectal adenomas. CA 34:167-176.

Luk GD, Baylin SB (1984). Ornithine decarboxylase as a biologic marker in familial colonic polyposis. NEJM 311:80-83.

McGregor DB, Jones RD, Karlin DA, Romsdahl MM (1982), Trophic effects of gastrin on colorectal neoplasms in the rat. Annals of Surgery 195(2):219-223

Moertel CG, Bargen JA, Dockerty M (1958). Multiple carcinomas of the large intestine: Review of the literature and a study of 261 cases. Gastroenterol 34:85-98.

Miller CH, Kussin SZ, Winawer SJ (1980), Characteristics of synchronous colonic polyps. Gastro Endosc 26:72.

Morson BC, Pang LSC (1967). Rectal biopsy as an aid to cancer control in ulcerative colitis. Gut 8:423-434.

Murray D, Hreno A, Dutton J, Hampson LG (1975). Prognosis in colon cancer: a pathologic reassessment. Arch Surg 110:908-913.

Papillon J (1980). The treatment of limited cancer of the rectum by intracavitary irradiation. Minerva Med 71: 763-765.

Podolsky DK, Isselbacher KJ (1984). Glycoprotein composition of colonic mucosa: specific alterations ulcerative colitis. Gastroenterol 87:991-998.

Reichmann A, Martin P, Levin B (1980). Double minutes in large bowel tumors. Gastroenterol 79:334-339.

Reilly JC, Rusin LC, Theuerkauf FJ (1982). Colonoscopy: its role in cancer of the colon and rectum. Dis Colon Rectum 25:532-538.

Riddell RH, GOldman H, RansohoffDF, Appelman HE, Fenoglio CM, Haggitt RC et al (1983). Dysplasia in inflammatory bowel disease: standardized classification with provisional clinical application. Human Path 14:931-968.

Riddell RH (1983). Dysplasia in inflammatory bowel disease, in pathology of the colon, small intestine and anus. In Norris HT (ed): "Churchill Livingstone" New York, NY, pp 95-97.

Sherlock P, Lipkin M, Winawer SJ (1980). The prevention of colon cancer. Am J Med 68:617-630.

Silverstein FE (1984). Research in gastrointestinal endoscopy. Gastrointest Endosc 30:267-268.

Stroehlein JR, Goulston K, Hunt RH (1984). An approach to evaluating the cause of a positive fecal occult blood test. CA 34:148-157.

Teague RH, Thornton JR, Manning AP, Salmon PR (1978) Colonoscopy for investigation of unexplained rectal bleeding. Lancet 1:1350-1351.

Tedesco FJ, Waye JD, Raskin JB et al (1978). Colonoscopic evaluation of rectal bleeding - a study of 304 patients, Ann Intern Med 89:907-909.

Tedesco FJ, Waye JD, Avella JR, Villalobos MM (1980). Diagnostic implications of the spacial distribution of colonic mass lesions (polyps and cancers): A prospective colonoscopic study. Gastrointest Endosc 26:95-97.

Tedesco FJ, Gottfried EB, Corless JK, Brownstein RE (1984). Prospective evaluation of hospitalized patients with nonactive lower intestinal bleeding - timing and role of barium enema and colonoscopy. Gastrointest Endosc 30:281-283.

Theoni RF, Menuck L (1977). Comparison of barium enema and colonoscopy in the detection of small colonic polyps. Radiology 124:631-635.

Warren S, Sommers SC (1949). Pathogenesis of ulcerative colitis. Am J Pathol 25:657-679.

Waye JD, Frankel A, Braunfeld SF (1980). The histopathology of small colon polyps. Gastrointest Endosc 26:80.

Williams AR, Balasooriya BA, Day DW (1982). Polyps and cancer of the large bowel: A necropsy study in Liverpool. Gut 23:835-842.

Williams CB, Hunt RD, Loose H (1974). Colonoscopy in the management of colon polyps. Br J Surg 61:673-682.

Williams CB Macrae FA, Bartram CI (1982). A prospective study of diagnostic methods in adenoma follow-up. Endoscopy 14:74-78.

Winawer SJ (1980). Screening for colorectal cancer: An overview. CA 45:1093-1098.

Carcinoma of the Large Bowel and Its Precursors, pages 133–149
© **1985 Alan R. Liss, Inc.**

THE AIR CONTRAST BARIUM ENEMA - INDICATIONS AND VALIDITY

Gerald D. Dodd, M.D.
Professor and Head, Division of Diagnostic
    Imaging
M.D. Anderson Hospital and Tumor Institute
Houston, Texas   77030

The air contrast barium enema is frequently thought to be a recent development in diagnostic radiology. This perception is incorrect. Detailed descriptions of both the single and double-contrast methods of examination were first published in 1911 (Haenisch) and 1923 (Fischer), respectively. Subsequently, in 1932, Gershon-Cohen and Shay advocated use of the double-contrast technique as "an additional routine examination to the barium enema" and, in 1949, Moreton and Yates described it as "the ideal routine study". Then as now there was resistance to this view; Garland (1949), for example, considered the technique to be of value in only 2-5% of patients. The major drawbacks cited include added discomfort and hazard for the patient, the added time and effort required to perform and interpret the examinations, excessive false-positive rates (polyps) and the apparent inability of the double-contrast enema to clearly identify some lesions which are obvious on single-contrast examinations. To the radiologist experienced in double-contrast methodology these objections are, in the majority, manifestations of improper technique and inexperience. The potential of the double-contrast enema has been well demonstrated by Welin and Welin (1976) who have shown that the majority of colon neoplasms, both benign and malignant, can be diagnosed by the technique. In their experience lesions between 0.5 and 1 cm can be detected routinely and the properly performed examination will include many neoplasms 2-3 mm in diameter. Needless to say, accuracy of this magnitude depends upon the proper performance of all aspects of the examination.

PREPARATION

The key to any adequate colonic examination is thorough preparation. The problem is complex from both the physiologic and pharmacologic standpoints. Nevertheless, if a few basic principles are followed, an adequate preparation can usually be obtained. Unquestionably, it is of value to maintain the patient on a low residue or liquid diet for at least 18 to 24 hours prior to examination. Oral hydration is extremely important since it prevents absorption of moisture from the stool and permits a more satisfactory response to a laxative.

The laxative or laxatives chosen should be reasonably potent. At the University of Texas M.D. Anderson Hospital and Tumor Institute we have for some years employed the preparation developed by Brown (1968) (Fig. 1). While there is no clear evidence that this regimen is superior to all others, it has been quite satisfactory in the majority of adults (Present, Dodd et al 1982). The sequence begins with a low residue diet starting at noon the day prior to examination. Hydration with oral liquids is begun concurrently and is continued until the time of the examination. A combination of laxatives is employed, including an initial saline cathartic for bulk evacuation (magnesium citrate) followed by a contact irritant (Bisacodyl). A 2000 cc tap-water enema is given in the Department of Diagnostic Radiology at least 45 minutes prior to the contrast study. The latter is essential to the performance of quality studies.

COLON PREPARATION

1. 18-hour Preparation Beginning at Noon

    A. Hydration - 10 - 12 glasses H_2O or juice over period of preparation.

    B Minimal low residue diet

    C. 8:00 p.m. - Magnesium Citrate (11 oz.)

    D. 10:00 p.m. - Bisacodyl, 5mg (4 tabs.)

2. 2000 cc Tap Water Enema - 45 minutes before examination.

Fig. 1.

CONTRAST MEDIA

There is a difference between the barium mixtures required for single-contrast studies and those utilized for double-contrast enemas. In the former a relatively dilute solution is necessary to permit penetration of the opaque column by the incident x-ray beam. In double-contrast enemas the primary requirement is for uniform coating of the bowel wall without flocculation or flaking of the thin layer of barium. The coating suspension must be considerably more viscid than the barium used for single-contrast studies, preferably on the order of an 85% weight-volume mixture. Because of the increased visocosity, relatively large bore enema tips and tubing are required.

It must be emphasized that the double-contrast procedure cannot be used as an appendage to the single-contrast examination. The coating of the mucous membrane produced by the type of barium used for single-contrast studies is inadequate for double-contrast examinations. Conversely, the high density of the suspension intended for double-contrast studies does not permit adequate penetration of the barium column for single-contrast examinations. So-called biphasic procedures have been recommended, however, for redundant sigmoid segments (de Roos 1984).

In recent years liquid premixed bariums have been marketed. The use of a standard water supply obviates many of the problems previously experienced in obtaining adequate suspensions and permits uniformity of examinations, not only in the same institution, but from community to community.

The quantity of air required will vary with the individual examination, but for practical purposes a total of 2500 cc is required for the average adult. If desired, the patient's discomfort can be minimized by the use of intravenous glucagon (1mg). However, this has the disadvantage of permitting flooding of the terminal ileum and most patients can adapt to distension of the bowel if the air is administered in an incremental fashion. For practical purposes glucagon does not significantly increase the sensitivity and specificity of the double-contrast examination and should only be used in selected instances such as great discomfort, spasm, suspected inflammatory disease, etc. (Thoeni et al 1984).

TECHNIQUE

The kilovoltage employed for double-contrast studies is usually considerably lower than for the single-contrast examination. Ninety kilovolts will usually ensure reasonably short exposure times while providing maximum radiographic contrast.

It is essential that thorough radiographic coverage of the bowel wall be obtained. This can only be achieved by making multiple films in multiple projections. The redundancy and circular nature of the bowel requires a sufficient number of projections to assure that the entire circumference to the lumen is visualized in profile as well as enface. If this is not done, the presence of small lesions cannot be excluded and, indeed, some very large masses may be overlooked due to superimposition of loops or puddling of barium (Fig. 2). Rosengren (1977) concluded that a minimum of 10 films per examination is necessary to provide complete coverage.

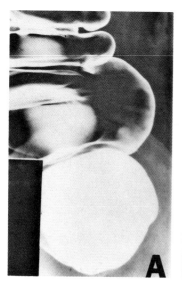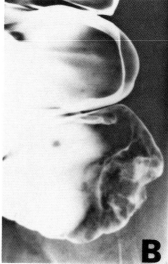

Fig. 2

Fig. 2. Effect of position on the visualization of intraluminal lesions. A. In the anteroposterior projection
there is no apparent abnormality of the cecum. B. In the
Trendelenburg position redistribution of the barium and
air permits visualization of a carcinoma of the cecal tip.

Minimum coverage requires 14 x 17 films of the
abdomen in the prone, supine, erect and lateral decubitus
projections. Of these the lateral, decubitus and erect
films are probably the most important since the dependent
position of the barium permits inspection of the majority
of the bowel wall without loss of detail due to excessive
amounts of barium (Fig. 3). Oblique films may be useful
on occasion, but are not essential and should be omitted
in younger patients to minimize the quantity of radiation
received.

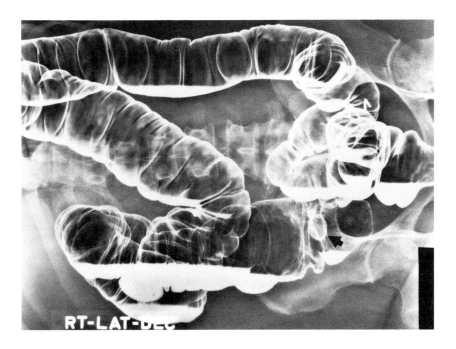

Fig. 3. Right lateral decubitus projection. The size and
distribution of the barium pool is readily determined.
There is a small lipoma of the cecum (arrow).

Also of importance are the lateral and angled projections of the rectum and sigmoid. The latter are made in both the supine and prone projections with the tube angled 30° cephalad and caudad respectively. The projections provide excellent coverage of the rectosigmoid and usually permit adequate visualization of the entire segment.

The double-contrast method does not negate the need for spot films made under fluoroscopic control. Oblique films of all flexures and redundancies are essential and should be made in both the erect and supine positions. The manipulation of the patient often serves to displace intraluminal artifacts and literally provides step-by-step coverage of the mucosal surface.

DIAGNOSTIC CRITERIA

The double-contrast barium enema is intended to disclose abnormalities of both the mucosal surface and the colonic outline. While changes in contour or well-defined filling defects can be demonstrated by the single-contrast high-kilovoltage method, minor alterations are best appreciated when visualization of the mucosal surface is possible. The aphthoid ulcerations of Crohn disease are readily recognizable by double-contrast examination, but since they do not necessarily alter the margins of the bowel wall, they may not be apparent on the single-contrast study (Fig. 4). The same is true of the granular mucosal pattern and superficial ulcerations characteristic of early ulcerative colitis (Fig. 5). Similar considerations apply to other forms of inflammatory bowel disease.

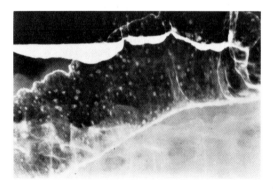

Fig. 4.

Fig. 4. Aphthoid ulcerations of Crohn disease (right lateral decubitus projection). The ulcerations are confined to the mucous membrane and do not alter the contours of the bowel.

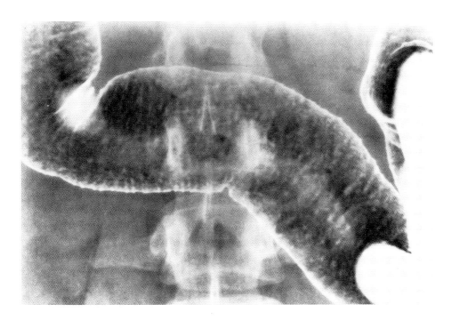

Fig. 5. Acute ulcerative colitis There are multiple, evenly distributed superficial ulcerations as compared with the random distribution in Crohn disease.

The radiologic signs of carcinoma of the colon are well-known and consist primarily of mass and mucosal destruction. Cancers of this type may be overlooked due to faulty preparation or technical error, but are readily diagnosed with a properly performed study of either the single or double-contrast variety. More important is the demonstration and classification of small polypoid tumors. If benign, no treatment other than observation or colonoscopic removal may be necessary. On the other hand, the malignant types offer the best opportunity for cure and reasonably reliable diagnostic criteria have been developed. Youker et al (1968) consider the following criteria to be of importance.

1. Size

The probability of malignancy increases with size. Less than 5% of tumors under 1 cm in diameter are malignant whereas approximately one-third of those between 1 and 2 cm and two-thirds of those larger than 2 cm are malignant.

Virtually all polyps under 3 mm in size are of the hyperplastic variety and have no malignant potential. Exceptions may be found in the polyps associated with the early stages of familial polyposis and Gardner syndrome. These are true adenomas and a malignancy will eventually supervene if the large bowel is not removed. (Fig. 6).

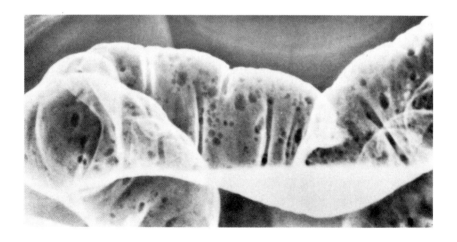

Fig. 6. Gardner syndrome (right lateral decubitus projection). All defects represent true adnomas.

2. Base Configuration

In general, if the width of polypoid mass exceeds its height, the probability of malignancy is increased (Fig. 7).

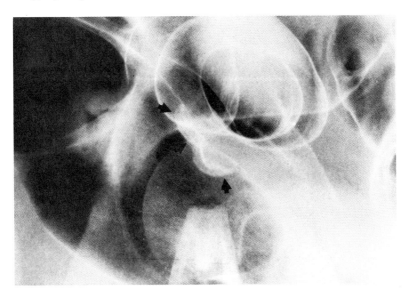

Fig. 7. Plaque-like carcinoma of the anterior rectal wall. The base of the polypoid mass is approximately twice its maximum height.

3. Indented Base

Notching of the base implies invasion of the wall of the bowel and is applicable only to broad-based polypoid masses (Fig. 8): pedunculated polyps may show an indentation related to traction.

4. Pedicle Formation

The incidence of malignancy in polyps with a well-defined pedicle is extremely small (Fig. 9).

The filform polyps associated with chronic inflammatory bowel disease have no malignant potential (Fig. 10).

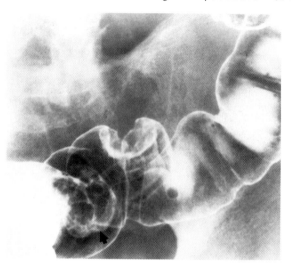

Fig. 8. Small carcinoma of the sigmoid colon   There is
irregular notching of the base. A large, adenomatous
sentinal polyp is also present (arrows).

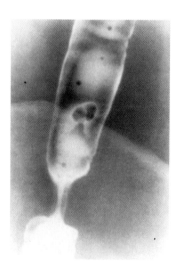

Fig. 9. Pedunculated tubular adenoma of the descending
colon. Polyps with a well-defined stalk are seldom
malignant.

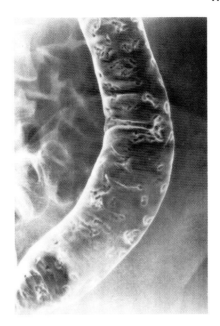

Fig. 10. Inflammatory polyps of the descending colon in a patient with quiescent non-specific ulcerative colitis. These have no malignant potential.

5. Roughened Surface

An irregular surface is far more common in malignant than in benign masses. Approximately one-third of villous adenomas have a characteristic lace-like appearance (Fig. 11). Since the incidence of malignancy is approximately 8 times higher than in the more common tubular adenoma, recognition of the pattern is important. Unfortunately, only about one-third of villous adenomas show the "typical" roentgen appearance.

6. Growth Rate

The probability of malignancy in polyps which require 1200 or more days to double in size is on the order of 13%. With doubling times of less than 1200 days, the probability rises to 87%.

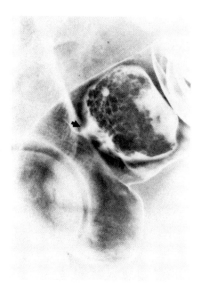

Fig. 11. Villous adenoma of the rectum. There is a broad, short stalk (arrows) and the head of the polyp shows a lace-like pattern. These tumors have a high malignant potential.

The significance of these findings when considered in toto is illustrated by the following:

1. The chances of a polyp being malignant are but 1:92 if the tumor is less than 1 cm in diameter, smooth on the surface and shows no indentation of the base.

2. If the tumor exceeds 2 cm in diameter, has a roughened surface and an indented base, the chances increase to 23:27.

RESULTS

Acceptance of the double-contrast enema as the primary radiologic method of examination of the colon has increased, but there is still debate as to the need or desirability for routine use of the procedure. Advocates of the single-contrast high-kilovoltage method contend that with careful fluoroscopy and spot filming the accuracy of the two techniques is approximately equal (Johnson et al 1983). Figiel (1969) has reported finding polyps in 7.5% of patients in the course of routine single-contrast examinations. By comparison Welin (1967), in a series of 36,000 consecutive air studies, found polyps in 12.5%, a rate which equaled the frequency of polyps found at autopsy in his institution. The 40% difference in the two series essentially reflects the incidence of polyps in the rectosigmoid region, an area difficult to examine by the single-contrast method. Similarly, Thoeni et al (1977) reported an error rate in the diagnosis of small colonic polyps of but 11.7% with double-contrast enemas as opposed to 45.2% with the single-contrast variety. Gelfand et al (1981) found the sensitivity of polyp detection with double-contrast studies to be 87% as compared to 59% for the single-contrast technique. de Roos et al (1984) have also reported a clear-cut superiority for double-contrast or biphasic examinations over the single-contrast technique in the detection of polyps over 1 cm in diameter, particularly in the sigmoid area.

It is our opinion that the double-contrast enema is the preferred means of examination. The technical aspects do differ from those of the single-contrast high-kilovoltage procedure and, due to differences in marginal contrast, the diagnostic criteria which apply to the conventional barium enema are not always transferrable to the double-contrast study. Nevertheless, the criteria are precise and, when properly used, can result in improved diagnostic efficiency due to the ability of the technique to detect minor changes in the mucous membrane.

There is a frequent misconception that the single-contrast examination is a more benign procedure than the double-contrast study. However, both require the same rigorous preparation. In our experience only toxic megacolon, severe hemorrhagic states, suspected perforation or acute and subacute obstructions are contraindications to the preparatory regimen and a definitive diagnostic procedure. There is some dispute on the wisdom of preparing the bowel of a patient with peridiverticulitis but unless there are overt signs of perforation, this is usually an acceptable proceeding.

The hazard of perforation has been over-emphasized. Diner et al (1981) have demonstrated that intracolonic pressure during a routine double-contrast study does not exceed that found in conventional examinations. Unquestionably, the double-contrast examination is more time consuming, but if it is accepted that a patient is deserving of the most sensitive and specific technique available, the double-contrast study is the procedure of choice.

In recent years there has been a tendency to resort to flexible proctosigmoidoscopy or colonoscopy without an antecedent barium enema. It is correctly claimed that direct visualization of the lumen of the bowel is the more accurate method of examination. However, the usual examination with a flexible 60 cm sigmoidoscopy costs $65 - $75 and only a portion of the colon is examined. Charges for complete colonoscopy range from $450 to $1,000 and visualization of the entire colon may not be achieved. Williams (1974), an experienced colonoscopist, has found that properly performed double-contrast examinations identify 98% of all colonoscopically visualized polyps greater than 1 cm in diameter and up to 95% of those more than 5 mm in diameter. Fort et al (1983), detected 98% of all colonic neoplasms more than 15 mm in diameter by double-contrast enema. They were able to predict malignancy in 90% and concluded that the probability of a patient with a negative double-contrast study being free of malignant tumor was approximately 99%.

Beggs et al (1983), detected 96% of colonic carcinomas on double-contrast barium enema examination and found this rate equal to that for colonoscopy in their institution. In both instances, the majority of mistakes occurred in the sigmoid colon. Similarly, Ott et al (1980), have found a false-negative rate of only 8.4% in the diagnosis of 190 polyps identified by colonoscopic examination. Again the primary source of difficulty was in the sigmoid segment.

The costs for the double-contrast examination vary between $95 and $125 and, since the methodology can be utilized in any hospital or private setting, the examination is within reach of the average patient and is an alternative screening method in high risk populations.

It is a mistake to consider colonoscopy and the double-contrast barium enema competitive examinations: the two methods are complimentary. Radiologic detection of a significant abnormality should be followed by colonoscopic verification and/or biopsy. This approach is advocated by Williams et al (1974) who routinely use some form of barium enema before colonoscopy.

It must be emphasized that the double-contrast enema requires meticulous attention to detail. The radiologist must not only assume responsibility for the technical preparation of the patient and the education of colleagues from other disciplines in the requirements of the procedure. However, if properly performed and interpreted, the double-contrast barium enema is cost-effective and can be depended upon to provide prompt and dependable information.

SUMMARY

The double-contrast barium enema is a highly accurate and readily available procedure which is capable of diagnosing benign and malignant disease of the colon at an early state. The level of accuracy is a function of the radiologist's knowledge and willingness to assume complete responsibility for the patient. While reasonable results may be obtained with the high-kilovoltage single-contrast method, it is our opinion that the double contrast examination is the more sensitive procedure and therefore the technique of choice.

The double-contrast examination ideally compliments the colonoscope and offers an alternative method for initial survey procedures or low cost follow-up examinations.

REFERENCES

Beggs I, Thomas BM (1983). Diagnosis of carcinoma of the colon by barium enema. Clinical Radiology 34:423.

Brown G (1968). The direct air contrast colon examination, A rapid simplified highly diagnostic procedure. Garland R. Brown, 1968. Scientific Exhibit at the American Roentgen Ray Society Meeting, San Francisco.

de Roos A, Hermans J, Odo Op den Orth J (1984). Polypoid lesions of the sigmoid colon: A Comparison of single-contrast, double-contrast, and biphasic examinations. Radiology 151:597.

Diner WC, Patel G, Texter EC Jr., Baker ML, Tune JM, Hightower MD (1981). Intraluminal pressure measurements during barium enema: Full column vs. air-contrast, AJR 137:217.

Figiel SJ (1969). Colon examination techniques, Proceedings of the First Standardization Conference - 1969. Detection of colon lesions, American College of Radiology ad hoc Committee on Detection of Cancer of the Colon, p 132.

Fischer AW (1923). A new Roentgenologic method for examination of the large intestine: A Combination of the contrast material enema and insufflation with air. (Originally in: Klin Wschr, 2:1595, August 20, 1923) Translation in: Classic Descriptions in Diagnostic Radiology, ed. Bruwer A, Vol 2, Charles C. Thomas P 1971.

Fork FT, Lindstrom C, Ekelund G (1983). Double-contrast examination in carcinoma of the colon and rectum. Acta Radiologica 24:Fasc 3, 177.

Garland H (1949). Quoted in: The Double Contrast Examination with the Welin Modification by Welin and Welin, p 2 - Thieme Edition/Publishing Sciences Group Inc. 1976.

Gelfand DW, Ott DJ (1981). Single vs double contrast gastrointestinal studies: critical analysis of reported statistics. AJR 137:523.

Gershon-Cohen J, Shay H (1932). The colon as studied by double-contrast enema. Am J Roentgen 27:838.

Haenisch GF (1911). The value of the roentgen ray in the early diagnosis of carcinoma of the bowel. Amer Quart Roentgenol 3:175.

Johnson CD, Carlson HG, Taylor WG, Weiland LP (1983). Barium enemas of carinoma of the colon: Sensitivity of double and single-contrast studies. AJR 140:1143.

Moreton RD, Yates CW (1949). Roentgenologic study of the colon: Value of the double-contrast enema. Tex S J Med 45:157.

Ott DJ, Gelfand DW, Wu WC, Kerr RM (1980). Sensitivity of double-contrast barium enema: emphasis on polyp detection AJR 135:327.

Present AJ, Jansson B, Burhenne HJ, Dodd GD, Goldberg HI, Goldstein HM, Miller RE, Nelson JA, Stewart ET (1982). Evaluation of 12 colon clearnsing regimens with single-contrast barium enema. AJR 139:855.

Rosengren JE (1977). Radiographic investigation of experimentally induced colonic tumors in the rat, Malmo General Hospital.

Thoeni RF, Menuck L (1977). Comparison of barium enema and colonoscopy in the detection of small colonic polyps. Radiology 124:631.

Thoeni RF, Vandeman F, Wall SD (1984). Effect of glucagon on the diagnostic accuracy of double-contrast barium enema examinations. Am J Roentgen 142:111.

Youker JE, Welin S, Main G (1968). Computer analysis in the differentiation of benign and malignant polypoid lesions of the colon. Radiology 90:794.

Welin S (1967). Results of the Malmo technique of the colon examinations. JAMA 199:119.

Welin S, Welin G (1976). The double-contrast examination of the colon. Experiences with the Welin modifications, Georg Thieme Verlag, Germany.

Williams CB Hung RH, Loose H, Riddell RH, Saki Y, Swarbrick FT (1974). Colonoscopy in the management of the colon polyps. Br J Surg 61:673.

Carcinoma of the Large Bowel and Its Precursors, pages 151–160
© 1985 Alan R. Liss, Inc.

ENDOSCOPIC LASER SURGERY

Randall W. Burt, M.D.   John H. Bowers, M.D.
John G. Hunter, M.D.   John A. Dixon, M.D.
Division of Gastroenterology, Department of
Medicine and the Department of Surgery
University of Utah School of Medicine
Salt Lake City, Utah 84132

INTRODUCTION

Laser energy is useful for medical applications because the tissue injury caused by this modality is very predictable (Fleisher et al 1983; Dixon 1983; Kelly et al 1980; Brown et al 1980). The area of injury is determined by the diameter of the laser beam striking the tissue surface. The depth of laser penetration into the tissue is dependent on the wavelength of laser light used. The type of tissue damage (i.e., coagulation, carbonization or vaporization) is related to the amount of energy applied to a given volume of tissue. Precise depth of penetration is especially important in the gastrointestinal tract where deep or erratic tissue damage may lead to bowel perforation. The Argon laser emits a wavelength which penetrates 1mm into gut tissues. It has therefore proved useful for treating superficial mucosal lesions of the stomach and bowel. The Neodymium;yttrium aluminum garnet (Nd:YAG) laser penetrates 4mm and is applied to deep and protuberant lesions. Argon and Nd:YAG lasers are especially suitable for gastrointestinal applications because the laser energy from both sources may be applied endoscopically through flexible quartz wave guides (Dixon 1983; Dixon et al 1982). This paper will describe our institution's laboratory and clinical experience with endoscopically directed Argon and Nd:YAG lasers in the gastrointestinal tract. Parameters of safety and efficacy for these lasers have been examined in both the dog model and the clinical setting. Results of this work will be presented.

ARGON LASER: Canine Experiments

A. Methods

Characteristics of the Argon laser were assessed in the canine colon by determining the depth of tissue injury at a single energy density, and by determining the time required to perforate with constant laser application (Dixon et al 1982). For the depth of penetration experiment, a laser energy density of 300 joules per square centimeter was achieved with a five second application of a two watt Argon laser to canine colon. The energy was applied with a quartz fiber inserted through a colonoscope. The tip of the fiber was held 5mm from the bowel surface. Fifteen lesions were created in this manner in the intact colon of each of five dogs.

The total time required to perforate the canine colon with Argon laser was determined next. Five dogs underwent colonoscopy and two watts of laser energy was directed through the quartz fiber. However, to simulate the worst possible clinical situation, the quartz fiber was held directly against the wall of the colon. The colon was inflated with CO_2, and laser energy was applied continuously until complete perforation was noted by viewing the colon through a laparotomy incision. A total of 53 perforations were created in the five dogs and the time to perforation was recorded.

B. Results:

In the depth of tissue injury studies, all 60 lesions examined eight days after laser application were completely healed. Of the 60 lesions examined four days after colonoscopy; 18 were completely healed, 20 showed injury to the submucosa only, 9 demonstrated injury through less than half of the muscularis, and 13 showed injury through greater than half of the muscularis. However, there were no perforations and peritonitis was not seen.

In the perforation studies, a mean time of 41±13 seconds was required to perforate the canine colon. The range was 20 to 100 seconds.

ARGON LASER: Human Studies

A. Methods:

After determination of the tissue effects in the experimental model, it was desired to study the affect of Argon laser at the same energy density on the human colon. An opportunity presented itself to study depth of penetration of injury in the human colon. A 50-year-old patient with Gardner's Syndrome who had undergone previous abdominal colonic resection and ileocolostomy required pelvic colectomy and ileostomy due to villous changes in several polyps. With informed consent of the patient and permission of the University Human Research Committee, fifteen 1-4mm sessile polyps were photocoagulated using the 2 watt Argon laser with output measured at the distal fiber tip. As in the dog studies, the laser was applied through a quartz fiber inserted through the biopsy channel of a flexible colonoscope. The tip of the quartz fiber was held 5mm distance from the mucosa creating a spot size of 2mm and the laser was applied for a duration of 5 seconds, giving an energy density of approximately 250 joules per centimeter squared. With some polyps, less than 5 seconds were used because of rapid blanching of the polyp. Because the treatment spot size was 2mm, polyps larger than this diameter required up to three sites of application. At the conclusion of treatment, each entire polyp appeared white but there was no carbonization, cavitation or vaporization. Four days after laser treatment the pelvic colon and rectum were excised. All 15 coagulated lesions were identified, fixed and stained with hematoxylin and eosin for determination of penetration of tissue injury.

After this depth of penetration study, eleven patients with Gardner's Syndrome, ileocolostomy and multiple polyps in the remaining colon were selected for laser treatment. There were six men and five women. The mean time since removal of the abdominal colon was ten years. All had undergone previous electrocoagulation of polyps (2-11 treatments). Two hundred and eleven 1-6mm polyps were photocoagulated at 18 treatment sessions in these patients. Lesions ranged in size from 1-6mm. All polyps larger than 3mm were biopsied and the location of each lesion was charted. The patients underwent endoscopy four days, twelve days, and three months after the initial application of the laser. Any additional polyps were photocoagulated at this time.

B. Results:

In the depth of penetration study, the surgical specimen revealed no gross evidence of serosal injury, peritonitis, or perforation. All lesions studied histologically demonstrated complete ablation of the mucosal polyp with no laser penetration beyond the submucosa. There was no muscularis penetration evident in any section. Coagulation of submucosal vessels was noted in most sections. In the clinical study no complications occurred in the Gardner's Syndrome patients who underwent Argon laser photoablation of colonic polyps. The mean time required per treatment session was 35 minutes; the mean number of polyps treated per session was 14; and the maximum number of polyps treated at one session was 41. Endoscopic examination of the photocoagulation sites four days following laser therapy showed that all treated polyps had sloughed leaving a healing superficial ulcer. Nearly all ulcers were healed at eight days and complete healing was present in all ablation sites at 12 days follow-up. Subsequent endoscopy revealed punctate of linear white scars at treatment sites.

Following the initial demonstration of safety and efficacy, the Argon laser was applied to several clinical situations which will be described later.

Nd:YAG LASER: Canine Studies

To study the tissue effects of Nd:YAG laser in the canine colon an experiment was designed to apply laser energy to this tissue at increasing energies and increasing duration of application. The tissue effects of various energy and time settings of the Nd:YAG laser were compared to the tissue effects of Argon laser and electrocautery. Nd:YAG laser and electrocautery energy sources produced deeper tissue injury than Argon laser. The depth of tissue injury for epithelial ablation was greatest with monopolar electrocautery, intermediate with Nd:YAG laser and least with Argon laser. A reasonable margin of safety between the energy needed for mucosal ablation and mucosal perforation was established for Nd:YAG laser.

CLINICAL APPLICATION OF ENDOSCOPIC LASER SURGERY

To date, 222 endoscopic laser procedures on 122 patients have been performed at our institution (Hunter et al, in press). Indications for laser surgical treatment can be divided into five categories: (1) Arteriovenous malformations; (2) active gastrointestinal hemorrhage: (3) benign mucosal lesions: (4) gastrointestinal cancer; and (5) anatomic anomalies. Success in these categories was defined as control of active gastrointestinal bleeding for greater than 24 hours, control of chronic bleeding or control of mucosal growths for greater than one month. Where available, a comparison of transfusion requirements before and after laser therapy was made in those patients with bleeding lesions. All procedures were performed by experienced endoscopists with a molectron model 8000 Nd:YAG laser and the HGM endo-8 Argon laser.

A summary of the procedures and results appears in Table 1.

Arteriovenous Malformations:

Forty patients with arteriovenous malformations underwent 72 applications of laser photocoagulation. Details of the patients treated are given in Table 1. Arteriovenous malformations were found in the stomach of 24 patients, in the duodenum of 7 patients, and in the colon of 15 patients. Four patients had hereditary hemorrhagic telangectasia. Concomitant diagnoses in the remainder included 12 patients with aortic stenosis and three patients with renal failure. Procedures were judged to be successful in 36 patients (90%), intermediate in three patients (7%), and a failure in one patient (3%). There were no complications. However, three deaths, all related to cardiac and renal failure, occurred within one month of treatment. Transfusion requirements were decreased from an average of 17 ± 5.9 units per patient in the year phototherapy to 1 ± 0.8 units in the year after phototherapy ($p<0.01$).

TABLE 1

SUMMARY OF 222 GASTROINTESTINAL ENDOSCOPIC LASER PROCEDURES PERFORMED AT THE UNIVERSITY OF UTAH BETWEEN 12/1/77 AND 9/1/83

	Arteriovenous Malformations	Active GI Bleeding	Benign Mucosal Lesions	GI Cancer	Anatomic Anomalies
No. of Patients	40	45	17	14	6
No. of Procedures	72	56	38	45	11
Mean Age	67	62	43	66	58
(range)	(33–87)	(21–87)	(19–82)	(33–90)	(29–87)
Sex: Male	21	29	7	12	4
Female	19	16	10	2	2
Endoscopic Procedure					
EGD	53	53	2	15	11
Flex Sig	1	2	33	29	–
Colonoscopy	13	–	3	1	–
General Result of Laser Phototherapy					
Success	36 (90%)	37 (82%)	13 (76%)	12 (86%)	4 (66%)
Indeterminate	3 (7%)	–	3 (18%)	1 (7%)	1 (17%)
Failure	1 (3%)	8 (18%)	1 (6%)	1 (7%)	1 (17%)
Operative Mortality	3 (7%)	6 (13%)	–	4 (28%)	–

Active Gastrointestinal Bleeding:

Forty-five patients underwent 56 laser phototherapy sessions for control of gastrointestinal bleeding. Bleeding sources included peptic ulcer, 19 patients; esophageal varices, 13 patients; gastritis, 4 patients; Mallory-Weiss tear, 3 patients; benign tumor, 2 patients; postoperative bleeding, 4 patients. Nd:YAG laser was used on 52 occasions and Argon laser on 5 occasions. Complications included aspiration pneumonitis in 3 patients, pleural effusion in 2 patients, cardiac arrest in 2 patients, and increased bleeding in 6 patients. Six patients died within one month of laser treatment of causes unrelated to the laser therapy. Control of bleeding was achieved initially in 37 (82%) patients; however, rebleeding occurred in 4. In 3 of these bleeding was cvontrolled with a seond endoxcopy. Control of bleeding was not achieved initially in 8 patients. In 2 of these, control of bleeding occurred during a second photocoagulation attempt. The other 6 patients went to laparotomy for control of bleeding.

Benign Mucosal Lesions:

Seventeen patients underwent 38 endoscopic laser procedures for ablation of benign mucosal lesions. Eleven of the 17 patients had Gardner's syndrome or familial polyposis coli and had previously undergone subtotal colectomy with ileorectal anastamosis. These patients were already being seen routinely for rectal surveillance and monopolar electrocautery polypectomy. During laser therapy sessions, biopsies were taken of polyps over 4mm and then all polyps were treated with Argon laser. Over 500 small sessile adenomatous polyps have been treated without complication on an outpatient basis. In ten patients polyp growth has been controlled with periodic treatment. One patient has required proctectomy for aggressive mucosal dysplasia. None of the patients have developed malignancy during therapy.

The Argon laser has also been used for photoablation of sporadic sessile colonic adenomatous polyps in 2 patients, gastric polyps in one patient and Barrett's esophagus in one patient. Standard treatment for these lesions were considered difficult or associated with excessive risk in each of these 4 patients. To date, short term follow-up (4 months to one year) has demonstrated no recurrence of lesions. Three patients with rectal bleeding from endometriosis coli have undergone Nd:YAG laser photocoagulation for destruction of the ectopic endometrial tissue. Although laser phototherapy reduced rectal bleeding in this group, the benefit was only partial and lasted only until the appearance of more endometrial implants. There have been no complications or mortality in the patients treated for benign mucosal lesions.

Gastrointestinal Cancer:

Fourteen patients have undergone 45 procedures for gastrointestinal cancer palliation. Nd:YAG laser has been used on 38 occasions, Argon laser on 6 occasions, and a combination on one occasion. Cancers treated included carcinoma of the esophagus, 4 cases; gastric carcinoma, one case; adenocarcinoma of the small bowel, one case; colorectal carcinoma, 7 cases; malanoma of the GI tract, one case; and colangiocarcinoma, one case. In patients with metastatic disease or those presenting a prohibitive operative risk, indications for laser surgical intervention included obstruction, 4 cases; bleeding, 5 cases; and local control, 6 cases. Thirteen of 14 patients were successfully palliated with one to 6 Nd:YAG phototherapy sessions. All patients completing the photoablation protocol were free from obstruction or hemorrhage at the time of death. The overall mortality of this group was 28% at one month and 64% at 4 months follow-up. The only complication of laser therapy was a transient episode of bleeding following laser photovaporization of an esophageal neoplasm. There were no perforations or mortality caused by endoscopic laser phototherapy.

Anatomic Anomalies:

Six patients have undergone 11 endoscopic laser procedures for incision of anatomic anomalies. Three of these patients had benign esophageal stricture (one had an esophageal web, one had a Schatzki's ring, and one had an anastomotic redundancy). All of these patients failed bouginage treatment but were relieved by Nd:YAG incision. Two patients with vomiting following gastric partitioning underwent stomal incision and dilation with Nd:YAG laser. This was only partially successful in one patient. Finally, one patient with multiple pancreatic pseudocysts compressing the posterior wall of the stomach underwent endoscopic Nd:YAG laser mediated incision and drainage of the pseudocyst. Complete resolution of the pseudocyst resulted. There was no morbidity or mortality in this group.

CONCLUSION:

In summary, canine and human studies were undertaken to quantitate the safety and efficacy parameters of endos-copically directed Argon and Nd:YAG lasers in the bowel. These lasers have been applied to several clinical gastrointestinal problems. The success of endoscopically applied lasers in these situations has been encouraging. Control of hemorrhage in both acute and chronic gastro-intestinal bleeding problems has been achieved. Unresect-able bowel tumors have been palliated and benign tumors which could not be resected by standard methods have been ablated. The primary use of endoscopically directed lasers to treat neoplastic bowel lesions is limited by the inability to judge the extent and histology of the lesion with these ablative procedures. Nonetheless, when removal or palliation cannot be accomplished by standard methods, laser phototherapy appears to be a promising alternative.

REFERENCES

Bown SG, Salmon PR, Storey DW, Calder BM, Kelly DF, Adams N, Pearson H, Weaver BMQ (1980). Nd:YAG laser photocoagulation in the dog stomach. Gut 21:818-825.

Dixon JA, Burt RW, Rotering HR, McCloskey DW (1982). Endoscopic argon laser photocoagulation of sessile colonic polyps. Gastrointest Endosc 28:162-165.

Dixon JA (1983). Surgical application of lasers. Yearbook Medical Publications, Chicago, IL.

Hunter JG, Bowers JH, Burt RW, Sullivan JJ, Stevens SL, Dixon JA. Lasers in endoscopic gastrointestinal surgery. Am J Surg (in press).

Kelly DF, Bown SG, Salmon PR, Calder BM, Pearson H. Weaver BMQ (1980). The nature and extent of biological changes induced by argon laser photocoagulation in canine gastric mucosa. Gut 22:1047-1055.

Therapeutic Laser Endoscopy in Gastrointestinal Diseases. Editors, Fleisher D, Jensen D, Bright-Asary P. Martinus Nijhoff, Boston, 1983. Chapters 1 and 2.

Carcinoma of the Large Bowel and Its Precursors, pages 161–173
© 1985 Alan R. Liss, Inc.

ANIMAL MODEL FOR COLORECTAL CANCER

Norman D. Nigro, M.D.
Clinical Professor of Surgery
Wayne State University School of Medicine
Detroit, Michigan 48226

INTRODUCTION

An animal model is an important part of the armamentarium of cancer researchers. While some forms of the disease occur spontaneously in animals, cancer of the intestine is rare. Furthermore, its effective induction by artificial means is a recent development. Lorenz in 1941 found that methylcholantrene given orally to mice caused cancer of the large intestine, but the incidence was low (Lorenz, Stewart 1941). Later, Walpole discovered that derivatives of aminobiphenyl induced intestinal cancers in some rats (Walpole 1952). Spjut injected rats with a high dose of 3,2'-dimethyl-4-aminobiphenyl daily for prolonged periods and found that 33% of the animals developed tumors of the large intestine, predominantly adenomas (Spjut, Noall 1970). However, the rats also developed a number of other benign and malignant tumors, in fact 64% of the female rats developed tumors in the breast. Therefore, it had limited value for the study of intestinal cancer, and an animal model was not widely used until after 1968.

Laqueur and Spatz were studying the neurotoxic effects caused by the ingestion of cycasin when in 1962 they discovered that animals fed the substance for 6 or 7 months developed multiple cancers of the intestine in addition to cancers in the liver and kidneys (Laqueur, Spatz 1968). Laqueur became interested in this carcinogenic effect and did several important studies which led to the discovery of the carcinogens currently used to study intestinal cancer in animals (Laqueur 1965).

CURRENT ANIMAL MODEL

Once the carcinogenicity of cycasin was established, studies were undertaken to find its active metabolite, and then to synthesize it in order to make it available for general use since the plant product was in short supply. The active metabolite in cycasin was found to be the glucoside of methylazoxymethanol. Matsumoto sythesized the compound, methylazoxymethanol acetate (MAM) which Laqueur found to be an even more effective intestinal carcinogen for rats than cycasin. Unlike cycasin, it was effective when given parenterally and was active in germ-free animals.

Druckrey and associates then investigated the carcinogenicity of two related compounds, 1,2-dimethylhydrazine (DMH) and azoxymethane (AOM) (Druckrey 1970). They found them to be effective, highly specific intestinal carcinogens for rats. Virtually all the animals developed multiple cancers of the large intestine plus an occasional cancer of the ear canal. They were most effective when given subcutaneously, but were also active when administered by stomach tube.

Of the three carcinogens, MAM. DMH and AOM; DMH is used most frequently and it is generally given subcutaneously, the average dose being 15 mg/kg once a week. Lower doses are less effective, while larger doses increase tumor yield. Multiple doses produce a cumulative tumor yield with a shorter latency period. Azoxymethane is similar to but slightly more potent than DMH. The average dose is 8 mg/kg. We have found that eight weekly injections are as effective as 26 weekly doses (unpublished material). Methylazoxymethanol acetate is not as effective as DMH or AOM, so the dose is about twice that of DMH. A single injection of any one of these compounds will induce intestinal cancer, a fact important in studies of the different phases of carcinogenesis.

Direct-acting colon carcinogens are also available as first shown by Narisawa et al (Narisawa et al 1971, 1976). Intrarectal instillation of N-methyl-N'nitro-N-nitrosoquanidine (MNNG, 2 mg. twice a week) or methylnitrosourea (MNU, 2 mg/week) results in the formation of tumors in that portion of the colon exposed to these chemicals. These two carcinogens are effective in several species of rodents, including guinea pigs which are resistant to the hydrazine derivatives.

EXPERIMENTAL ANIMALS

Since spontaneous neoplasms of the intestinal tract are rare in most animals, especially rodents, and since we have good, organ specific carcinogens that are effective in rats and mice, chemically induced neoplasms represent a particularly useful model for the study of colon cancer. It is important to note that among rodents there are species and strain differences in the degree of susceptibility to the carcinogens. Rats and mice are used most frequently, and several studies describing strain differences have been published (Diwan, Blackman 1980). In this country, Sprague-Dawley is the most susceptible strain of rats and therefore is used more often than any other variety.

Anatomical alterations of the intestinal tract can be used to develop useful information on the process of cancer formation in rats and mice. The following are examples of those that have been reported: (a) resection of the distal part of the small intestine causes a compensatory hyperplasia of the mucosa of the large intestine (Oscarson et al 1979). (b) A segment of large intestine can be placed in the small intestinal circuit and vice versa (Gennaro et al 1973). This, of course, exposes the large intestine to the small intestinal environment and the small intestine to the fecal stream of the colon, an alteration which evaluates the importance of luminal factors. (c) Colostomies can be done to defunctionalize the large intestine distal to the colostomy site (Campbell et al 1975). This removes the fecal stream from the large bowel beyond that point. The same effect also can be achieved by isolating a loop of large bowel attaching each end to the skin while joining together that which remains to reestablish intestinal continuity (Rubio, Nylander 1981). The excluded loop has viable mucosa which can be studied directly in several ways. (d) Finally, the bile duct of the rat can be divided at its junction with the intestine near the outlet of the stomach and joined to the small intestine at a more distal site (Chomchai et al 1974). The effect is to increase the amount of bile that enters the large intestine. Naturally, other operative procedures are possible.

In designing a tumorigenesis study in animals, one must estimate as accurately as possible the degree of cancer challenge needed to show the effect of any single experimental factor. Cancer challenge can be moderated by the choice of carcinogen, its dosage, route of administration, and the number of applications. It can be altered by dietary factors. For example, a high fat diet increases the tumorigenic effect of most carcinogens. On the other hand, the addition of a bulking fiber such as wheat bran to the diet has an inhibitory effect provided the fat content is not also excessive (Nigro et al 1979). Finally, since different strains of animals vary in this susceptibility to intestinal carcinogens, the choice of the animal is an important consideration in the design of an experiment.

PATHOLOGY OF TUMORS

Azoxymethane or its related compounds induce intestinal cancers primarily in the proximal small intestine and in all sections of the large intestine although tumors generally are more numerous in the distal half of the colon. Their number, size, distribution, and the degree of differentiation are related to the amount and number of doses of the carcinogen. Grossly and microscopically, the tumors resemble adenocarcinomas in humans. Animal tumors also penetrate the bowel wall and metastasize to regional lymph nodes and to the peritoneal cavity. Occasionally, cancers in animals metastasize to the liver and lung, but this is much less frequent than in humans (Ward et al 1973).

CARCINOGENESIS

The development of cancer is a long, multistep process. This was first demonstrated in mouse skin (Berenblum 1941), but later it was shown to be true in other organs, including the large intestine. The first stage, called initiation, is a rapid process which permanently damages the DNA of the cell. Promotion, the second stage, is a long phase that completes the transformation process begun by initiation. The mechanism of promotion is unknown, but all promoting factors cause chronic tissue damage which increases cell proliferation. Promoting agents alone will not cause cancer, and all hyperplastic sub- stances are not promotors. When considering prevention, promotion rather than initiation may be the crucial step. This is because initiation occurs quickly and appears to be difficult, if not impossible, to prevent. On the other hand, promotion requires repeated exposure to the promoting agent, and it takes a long time for completion. Hence, there is a significant time frame during which the carcinogenic process can be interrupted.

STUDIES SUPPORTING ADENOMA-CARCINOMA SEQUENCE

Most pathologists and surgeons believe that the majority of cancers of the large intestine in humans develop from adenomas. Morson has published evidence which suggests that large adenomas have a greater risk of developing cancer than small ones, and that villous adenomas which are multicentric in origin are more likely to become malignant than the more common tubular adenomas (Morson 1974).

Hill has developed an interesting hypothesis to explain the development of cancer from adenomas. He suggests that there are different factors responsible for each step in the formation of cancer from adenomas. One factor causes small adenomas to form from adenoma-prone mucosa. Another factor is responsible for the growth of small adenomas to large ones. Finally, a third factor transforms large adenomas to carcinomas (Hill 1980).

Animal studies lend some support to this hypothesis. For example, carcinogens can induce intestinal adenomas and/or carcinomas depending upon circumstances. Weak carcinogens generally induce benign lesions whereas strong ones cause only malignant tumors. Spjut found that rats injected with 3,2'dimethyl-4-aminobiphenyl (DMAB) developed intestinal tumors, most of which were benign adenomas, with only an occasional carcinoma (Spjut, Noall 1970). The incidence of all intestinal tumors in these animals was only about 30%. This suggests that DMAB is a weak intestinal carcinogen. Unfortunately, these studies failed to show any direct relationship between adenomas and carcinomas.

Narisawa et al conducted an interesting study instilling MNNG into the rectum of rats in a single dose followed by repeated injections of one or the other of two bile acids (Narasawa et al 1974). This direct-acting carcinogen induced both adenomas and carcinomas in that part of the large intestine exposed to the solution. With MNNG alone, only 25% of the animals developed tumors which were evenly divided between adenomas and carcinomas. The addition of multiple doses of bile acids increased the tumor yield at least twofold, but there were more benign lesions than malignant lesions. However, a few tumors contained both benign and malignant tissue. This correlates with the situation in humans, that is, some benign adenomas have areas of malignant degeneration.

The hydrazine group of compounds, DMH, AOM, MAM, are potent intestinal carcinogens. When administered to a susceptible strain of rat at an average dose schedule, all lesions are carcinomas. However, at low doses this is not so: For example, Ward conducted a study in male Fischer rats given a single subcutaneous injection of AOM ranging from 0.8 to 5.1 mg/rat (Ward 1975). The rats were sacrificed 48 weeks after carcinogen administration. Those rats injected with 1.7 mg AOM developed 11 intestinal tumors, all benign; the group that received 3.4 mg developed 23 benign and 2 malignant intestinal tumors; while those receiving the highest dose developed 11 benign and 5 malignant tumors. These results clearly demonstrated that very small amounts of the carcinogen induced adenomas, but as the dose increased, the percentage of cancers increased.

More recently, Deschner et al (1979) carried out a dose response study using DMH in mice. They used various doses and schedules of DMH administration. The lowest dose was 2.5 mg/kg injected weekly for six weeks, and the highest was 20 mg/kg given for 26 weeks. The results showed that with increasing doses of DHM, (a) there was an increased yield and decreased latency period, (b) with repeated doses, there was a rapidly cumulative tumor yield, and (c) new tumors continued to form even long after DMH injections had terminated. They also found that when several tumors were present in the same animal, their sizes were graded rather than uniform.

Many studies have been published that show an increased yield of cancers of the large intestine in animals injected with DMH, AOM, or MAM, and fed a high fat diet compared to those on the same dose of carcinogen but fed a low fat diet. The high fat diet also increases the degree of anaplasia of the cancers and the incidence of metastases (Nigro et al 1979). This means that a specific dietary factor significantly altered the carcinogenic process, and it has been shown that this effect occurs during the promotional phase of tumorigenesis.

Raicht et al completed a study which showed that a dietary factor selectively affected intestinal adenomas (Raicht et al 1980). They fed rats β-sitosterol, a plant sterol, then treated the animals with intrarectal instillations of MNU. Fifty-four percent of the control animals (no β-sitosterol) developed tumors, with an average of 1.1 tumors per rat, while in 33% of the animals the β-sitosterol-treated group developed tumors, with an average of 0.44 tumors per rat. Microscopically, most lesions were adenomas, but there were four tumors that contained both adenomatous tissue and invasive carcinoma. Again, this is analogous to the human observation. The important point of this study is that the inhibitor prevented the formation of adenomas but not carcinomas. There were as many cancers in the experimental animals as in the controls. This suggests that it is possible to inhibit only one of the stages of cancer development.

Prostaglandin inhibitors also appear to have a selective inhibitory effect on intestinal neoplasms. It has been known since the early 1970's that indomethacin has antitumor activity (Sykes, Maddox 1972). Pollard and Luckert (1980) and Kudo et al (1980) found that indomethacin, administered orally, inhibited the development of cancer of the large intestine induced in rats by a variety of carcinogens. The evidence suggested that early lesions were more effectively inhibited than advanced cancers, and that the effect of the drug occurred during the promotional phase of carcinogenesis. Because indomethacin is somewhat toxic, especially to the small intestine, Pollard and associates substituted piroxicam for indomethacin and found that it had the same inhibitory effect but with no evidence of toxicity (Pollard, Luckert 1984). Based on these observations, Waddell treated four patients with familial polyposis with sulindac, a similar nonsteroid anti-inflammatory drug, and found a marked reduction in the number of adenomas in all 4 patients, 3 in the rectal stump of patients who had a colectomy and 1 in a patient with an intact colon (Waddell, Loughry 1983). This corroborates the similarity between the disease in the animal model and its human counterpart and the fact that the drug selectively inhibits adenomas and only well differentiated carcinomas.

These observations, conducted primarily in animal experiments, lend some support to Hill's hypothesis. In summary, the studies show that the same intestinal carcinogen is capable of inducing adenomas and carcinomas, and that weak carcinogens or low doses of strong carcinogens tend to induce adenomas or at least very early malignant lesions. However, strong carcinogens given in moderate amounts induce malignant lesions. At least two studies demonstrated lesions that consisted of both benign and malignant tissue. The fact that a high fat diet greatly increases the effect of a carcinogen suggests that dietary factors can be responsible for the growth of small polyps to large ones, and even for the conversion of large benign lesions to carcinoma.

It is interesting to speculate on the possible cause of the formation of adenomas from normal mucosa. As Hill points out, there is very little information on the incidence of adenomas in the human large intestine in countries that have a low incidence of cancer. There are two studies, one by Muto et al (1977) and the other by Correa et al (1972) which show that in low incidence countries (Japan and Columbia) adenomas do occur in the large intestine, but the majority are small. However, the few large adenomas that occur in low incidence countries have the same cancer potential as they do in high incidence areas. The striking difference between the two areas is the much greater incidence of large adenomas in the high cancer incidence countries. It would be helpful to have more information of this kind, but these observations do support the possibility that adenoma formation is caused by a genetic factor (Hill 1980). If that were true, adenomas would represent initiated cells which only progress to a malignant state through a sequence of promotional steps, all of which probably are due to environmental factors. Evidence derived from the animal model is consistent with this hypothesis.

ORNITHINE DECARBOXYLASE

There is strong biochemical evidence for the multi-step concept of carcinogenesis. An example is ornithine decarboxylase (ODC), the rate limiting enzyme for the formation of polyamines. It is present only in very small amounts in quiescent cells, but its activity is markedly increased in tissues exposed to hyperplastic stimuli which include growth factors and tumor promotors. In 1978, Buffkin et al found high levels of ODC activity in two types of animal tumors, an implanted, Walker 256 carcinoma, and a chemically induced cancer in rats. They suggested from their results that ornithine decarboxylase activity might serve as a biological marker of cancer. (Buffkin et al 1978).

Recently, Luk, Baylin (1984) found increased ODC activity in normal appearing mucosa in patients with familial polyposis and progressively higher levels in the polyps and in polyps showing an increased degree of anaplasia. They suggested that ODC determination in the mucosa might serve as a marker to identify patients that have familial polyposis before the development of adenomas. Sherlock and Winawer published an editorial in the same journal commenting on the paper but went a step further, suggesting the possibility that ODC activity in the mucosa of the large intestine might be a marker for identifying people at high risk for colo- rectal cancer (Sherlock, Winawer 1984).

Rozhin et al (1984) in our laboratory conducted ODC determinations in rats under a variety of circumstances, including animals on a high-fat diet and in those with AOM induced cancers of the large intestine. The enzyme levels were increased in animals on the high fat-diet and in the normal appearing mucosa of rats with intestinal cancer. Highest levels were found in the malignant tissue itself. The administrtion of difluoromethylornithine (DFMO), a specific inhibitor of ODC, not only reduced the enzyme activity in the intestine, but also reduced AOM induced cancers. Finally, these investigators found ODC activity in humans to be markedly increased in colorectal cancers over that in the normal appearing mucosa adjacent to the lesions. While only a few adenomas were included in the study, their ODC activity was elevated over that of the adjacent normal appearing mucosa but less than that in malignant tissue.

It is clear that these two studies done independently and published very recently add support to the idea suggested by Buffkin as long ago as 1978 that ODC activity may well be a useful marker of cancer and serve to identify people at high cancer risk. Human studies are justified and are undoubtedly under way to confirm this possibility.

SUMMARY

The development of a satisfactory rodent model for cancer of the large intestine began with the discovery by Laqueur and associates in 1962 that the plant product, cycasin (methylazoxymethanol glycoside), is a potent carcinogen for rodents. Soon after that, DMH, AOM, and MAM were found to be even more efficent intestinal carcinogens in rats. These three compounds, plus two direct acting carcinogens (MNNG, MNU) are used almost exclusively in current animal investigations. Although all these chemicals have some degree of activity in all rodents, they are most effective in rats. Various rat strains differ somewhat in susceptibility, Sprague-Dawley being the most sensitive to these carcinogens.

Cancers of the large intestine in the animal model resemble adenocarcinomas in humans, and they spread in a similar manner except that metastases to the liver and lung are very uncommon in animals. Animal studies support epidemiological and human experimental observations of dietary factors involved in colorectal cancer formation.

Most physicians believe that the majority of colorectal cancers develop from preexisting adenomas. Morson has shown that large adenomas and villous adenomas have a greater risk of developing cancer than small adenomas. Hill has theorized that there are different factors responsible for the formation of small adenomas from normal mucosa, for the growth of small to large adenomas, and for the development of cancer from large adenomas. Animal studies provide some support for this concept. Weak intestinal carcinogens tend to induce more benign adenomas than carcinomas. Very small doses of strong carcinogens also induce some adenomas and a few early polypoid intestinal cancers after a long latent period. Moderate to large amounts of DHM, for example, induce only malignant lesions even when these lesions are as small as 1 mm. These observations suggest a relationship between adenomas and carcinomas.

There is also biochemical evidence to support the staged progression of carcinogenesis. An example is the graded increases in ODC activity that occur in tissues undergoing tumorigenesis.

REFERENCES

Berenblum I (1941). The cocarcinogenic action of croton resin. Cancer Res 1:807.

Buffkin D, Webber M et al (1978). Ornithine as a possible marker of cancer. Cnacer Res 38:3225-3229.

Campbell RL, Singh DV, Nigro ND (1975). Importance of the fecal stream on the induction of colon tumors by azoxymethane in rats. Cancer Res 35:1369-1371.

Chomchai C, Bhadrachari N, Nigro ND (1974). The effect of bile on the induction of experimental intestinal tumors in rats. Dis Colon Rectum 17:310-312.

Correa P, Duque E, Cuello C, Haenszel (1972). Polyps of the colon and rectum in Cali, Colombia. Int J Cancer 9:86-96.

Deschner EE, Long FC, Maskens AP (1979). Relationship between dose, time, and tumor yield in mouse dimethyl-hydrazine-induced colon tumorigenesis. Cancer Lett 8:23-28.

Diwan BA, Blackman KE (1980). Differential suscepti-bility of 3 sublines of C57BL/6 mice to the induction of colorectal tumors by 1,2-dimethylhydrazine. Cancer Lett 9:111-115.

Druckrey H (1970). Production of colonic carcinoma by 1,2,dialkylhydrazines and azoxyalkanes, in "Carcinoma of the colon and antecedent epithelium, (W.J. Burdette, ed.), Charles C. Thomas Publisher, Springfield, IL. pp. 267.

Gennaro AR, Villanueva R, Sukonthaman Y, Vathanophos V, Rosemond GP (1973). Cheical carcinogenesis in transposed intestinal segments. Cancer Res 33:536-541.

Hill MJ (1980). The Aetiology of Colorectal Cancer, Recent Advances in Gastrointestinal Pathology. (Ed Wright), Saunders

Kudo T, Narisawa T, Abo S (1980). Antitumor activity of indomethacin on methylazoxymethanol induced large bowel tumors in rats. Gann 71:260-264.

Laqueur GL (1965). The induction of intestinal neoplasma in rats with the glycoside cycasin and its aglycone. Virchows ARch. Pathol. Anat 340:151-163.

Laqueur GL, Spatz M (1968). Toxicology of cycasin. Cancer Research, Vol. 28:2262-2267.

Lorenz E, Stewart HL (1941). Intestinal carcinoma and other lesions in mice following oral administrtion of 1,2,5,6-dibenzanthracene and 20-methylcholanthrene. J Natl Cancer Inst 1:17.

Luk G, Baylin SB (1984). Ornithine decarboxylase as a biological marker in familial colonic polyposis, NEJM 311:80-83.

Morson B (1974). The polyp cancer sequence in the large bowel. Proc Royal Soc Med 67:451-457.

Muto T, Ishikawa K, Kino I et al (1977). Comparative histological study of adenomas of the large intestine in Japan and England, with special reference to malignant potential. Disease Col and Rect 20(1):11-16.

Narisawa T, Magadia NE, Weisberger JH, Wynder EL (1974). Promoting effect of bile acids on colon carcinogenesis after intrarectal instillation of N-methyl-N-nitro-N-nitrosoguanidine in rats. J Natl Cancer Inst 53:1093.

Narisawa T, Sato T, Hayakawa M, Sakuma A, Nakano H (1971). Carcinoma of the colon and rectum of rats by rectal infusion of N-methyl-N'-nitro-N-nitrosoguanidine. Gann 63:231.

Narisawa T, Wong CO, Maronpot RR, Weisburger JH (1976). Large Bowel carcinogenesis in mice and rats by several intrarectal doses of methylnitrosourea and negative effect of nitrite plus methylurea. Cancer Res 36:505-510.

Nigro ND, Bull AW, Klopfer BA, Pak MS, Campbell RL (1979). Effect of dietary fiber on azoxymethane-induced intestinal carcinogenesis in rats. J Natl Cancer Inst 62:1097-1102.

Oscarson JEA, Veen HF, Ross JS, Malt RA (1979). Ileal re-section potentiates 1,2-dimethylhydrazine induced colonic carcinogenesis. Ann Surgery 503-508.

Pollard M, Luckert PH (1980). Indomethacin treatment of rats with dimethylhydrazine induced intestinal tumors. Cancer Treat Rep 64:1323-1327.

Pollard M, Luckert PH (1984). Effect of Piroxicam on primary intestinal tumors induced in rats by N-methylnitrosourea. Cancer Letters 25:117-121.

Raicht RF, Cohen BI, Fazzini EP, Sarwal AN, Takahashi M (1980). Protective effect of plant sterols against chemically induced colon tumors in rats. Cancer Res 40:403-405.

Rozhin J, Wilson P, Bull A, Nigro ND (1984). Studies on ornithine decarboxylase activity in the rat and human colon. Cancer Res (in press).

Rubio CA, Nylander G (1981). Further studies on carcinogenesis of the colon of the rat with special reference to the absence of intestinal contents. Cancer 48:951-953.

Sherlock P, Winawer S (1984). Are there markers for the risk of colorectal cancer? NEJM 311:118-119.

Spjut HJ, Noall MW (1970). Colonic neoplasms induced by 3,2'-dimethyl-4-amino-biphenyl, in: " Carcinoma of the Colon and Antecedent Epthelium, (W.J. Burdette, ed.), Charles C. Thomas Publisher, Springfield, IL, pp. 280-288.

Sykes JAC, Maddox IS (1972). Prostaglandin production by experimental tumours and effects of anti-inflammatory compounds. Nature New Biology 237:59-61.

Waddell W, Loughry R (1983). Sulindac for polyposis of the colon. J Surg Onco 24:83-87.

Walpole AL, Williams MHC, Roberts DC (1952). The carcinogenic action of 4-aminobiphenyl and 3:2'dimethyl-4-aminobinphenyl. Brit. J. Industr Med 9:255-263.

Ward JM (1975). Dose response to a single injection of azoxymethane in rats. Vet Pathol 12:165.

Ward JM, Yamamoto RS, Carolyn AB (1973). Pathology of intestinal neoplasms and other lesions in rats exposed to azoxymethane. J Nat Cancer Inst 51:1029-1039.

Carcinoma of the Large Bowel and Its Precursors, pages 175–186
© 1985 Alan R. Liss, Inc.

A MULTISTAGE MODEL FOR HUMAN COLON CARCINOMA DEVELOPMENT
FROM TISSUE CULTURE STUDIES

Eileen A. Friedman, Ph.D.
Memorial Sloan-Kettering Cancer Center
1275 York Avenue
New York City, New York   10021

There is much clinical and experimental evidence that
colon carcinoma in man evolves through a series of preneoplastic stages. Preneoplastic colonic cells have been
characterized in normal-appearing epithelium or "flat
mucosae" from patients genetically at risk to develop
colon cancer. These cells differ from normal colonic
epithelial cells by a delay in terminal differentiation
which leads to an enlargement of the zone of dividing
cells within the colonic crypt, a test tube-like hollow
cylinder roughly 50-60 cells deep (Lipkin et al 1983;
Lipkin 1984). These patients include those with familial
polyposis or Gardner's Syndrome and those without polyposis, but with a family history of first-degree relatives
with colon cancer. More advanced premalignant epithelial
cells compose adenomas or benign tumors. Adenomas are the
direct precursors of carcinomas, with those adenomas
classified as villous by histopathology having a much
greater probability of giving rise to a carcinoma than the
generally smaller and less aberrant-appearing tubular
adenomas (Muto et al 1975). Detailed study of the cells
within sectioned adenomas led to the conclusion that the
dysplastic cells within adenomas were the cell type
directly preceding carcinoma (Konishi and Morson 1982).
Therefore, at least five types of premalignant colonic
epithelial cells have been identified by a combination of
histopathology and clinical studies: grossly normal-
appearing cells displaying delayed terminal differentiation from genetically high-risk nonpolyposis patients,
aberrantly differentiating but non-tumor cells from
familial polyposis patients, and cells composing various

histologically classified adenomas: tubular adenoma cells,
villous adenoma cells, and dysplastic cells.

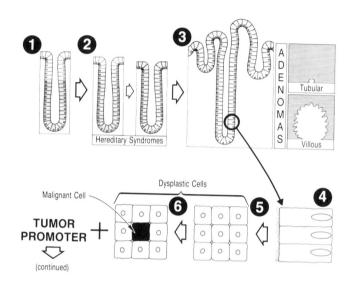

Figure 1. Multistage model of colon carcinoma in man

Figure 1 depicts ten distinct stages in the evolution
of colon carcinoma in man. In stage 1, the normal colonic
crypt appears diagrammatically in lengthwise section, with
the top of the crypt opening out into the gut lumen. Only
the epithelial cells are depicted, but not drawn to scale.
Their nuclei are attached to the basal part of the cell.
The filled-in areas in stages 1, 2, and 3 indicate the
fraction of the crypt in which dividing cells are found.
This is the lower two-thirds for the normal crypt, and is
enlarged in stages 2 and 3. Stages 2 left, 2 right, and 3
to 6 are hypothesized to occur after genetic changes,
probably mutagenesis of a stem cell. The nonmutagenic
effects of tumor promoters on dysplastic cells are shown
in stages 6 to 10. The area of replicating cells
increases in proportion to the terminally differentiated
area at the crypt top in stage 2, the hereditary
syndromes. Stage 2 left represents the nonpolyposis
high-risk groups and the right, the familial polyposis

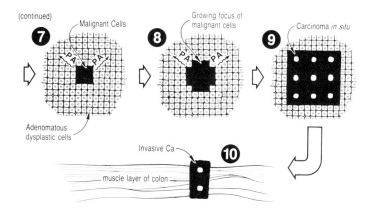

Figure 1 (continued)

flat mucosa.   No normal terminally differentiated cells
are indicated in stage 2 right because of the abnormal
fragility of the cells at the top of the crypt (Friedman,
et al 1984a) In stage 3, a lengthwise section of an adenoma is shown, all cell positions capable of containing a
dividing cell.   The abnormally lengthened crypts of the
adenoma are depicted as folding over on one another.   The
relative mean sizes of the tubular adenoma class and the
larger, on average, villous adenoma class is next depicted.   A section of adenoma cells with elongated nuclei is
shown in stage 4, enlarged relative to stages 1-3 to focus
on cellular changes.   One of these cells becomes mutated
and divides to form a focus of dysplasia, shown as a group
of multi-layered cells with central nuclei in stage 5.
This is an oversimplification of the adenoma to dysplasia
transition shown in detail in Friedman, Urmacher, Winawer
(1984b).   One of these dysplastic cells then becomes
mutated to carcinoma, the darkened cell in stage 6 shown
surrounded by dysplastic cells.   Growth of the focus of

carcinoma by continuous or pulsed secretion of plasminogen-activator (PA), with concomitant loss of the surrounding adenoma cells, is shown in stages 7 through 9. The carcinoma in situ in stage 9 finally expands to become an invasive carcinoma, two aberrant crypts of which are shown in cross-section invading through the muscle and fat layers of the colon in stage 10.

How do we know for sure that these premalignant cells fall into different classes? First, in sectioned tissue the cells composing adenomas are obviously less differentiated with little mucous when compared to normal colonic epithelial cells and cells from high-risk patients. Second, we have developed methods to place all of the premalignant cells and normal adult colonic epithelial cells in tissue culture. Differences in their properties are consistent with the categories stated, and will be discussed in detail.

The property which was most useful in differentiating the premalignant cell types was their differing response to the synthetic tumor promoter, TPA (12-0-tetradecanoyl-phorbol-13-acetate). Cells either displayed no discernible response, a mild proliferative response, or secreted the protease plasminogen activator which caused dramatic morphological changes in the cells. The effects of synthetic promoting agents on a wide variety of cultured cells have been reported, so what possible significance can these observations have to the in vivo progression of colon cancer? It may be useful to consider for a moment why tumor promotion has become used experimentally. Carcinogenesis originally began with an experimental animal and a putative carcinogen, and two questions were asked. Would the compound cause a tumor and, if so, where? This very necessary work simplified tumorigenesis into a one-step phenomenon. The introduction of promoting agents, which were initially observed to be cellular irritants, allowed tumor development to be broken up into stages and more closely approximate the multistage development of human cancer. A dose of a carcinogen too low to cause a tumor was selected. When this carcinogen was followed by repeated applications of a promoting agent, a tumor appeared. Either protocol alone did not give a tumor and reversing the order of application was ineffective. Effective carcinogens were mutagens, so an interpretation of the results was that a mutated cell was further modified by the promoting agent to become tumorigenic. A further improvement of the system using mouse skin in in vivo experiments has been described (Hennings et al 1983). A low dose of a mutagen followed by repeated applications of a promoter led to papillomas. A second mutagen than converted the papillomas to carcinomas. Experimental carcinogenesis was now divided into three stages.

Additional evidence suggests that tumor promotion has a relevance to human cancer development. It is not limited to skin carcinogenesis. TPA-mediated tumor promotion also occurs in the gastrointestinal tract (Goerttler et al 1979) and other organs (Blumberg et al 1984). This is not surprising as tumor promoters bind to a cellular receptor which is found on all nucleated vertebrate cells, including human cells (Blumberg et al 1984). This receptor has been identified as the enzyme, important in cellular regularion, protein kinase C (Nishizuka 1984). The tumor promoters somehow adventiously bind to and activate a normal cellular regulator and subvert its activity. Several structurally unrelated tumor promoters have been found (Sugimura 1982) which bind to this receptor protein. Diacylglycerol is at this time the only known endogenous compound which binds to and activates protein kinase C, but other endogenous-promoting agents may exist in the body.

The animal studies thus far suggest promoting agents somehow modify mutated and thus early-stage premalignant cells so that they become able to progress by further mutagenesis. The receptor studies demonstrate that all human cells, except red blood cells, could potentially be promoted so every human cancer could contain promotion stages in its evolution. The contribution of our laboratory has been to demonstrate that (1) premalignant human cells respond to promoting agents when placed in short-term primary culture; (2) dependent on the stage of the premalignant cell, the response to promoting agents differed; (3) the differing responses could be used to order the different premalignant cells described above into a sequence between normal cells and carcinoma cells; (4) experimental evidence exists for the role of promoting agents at different stages in the premalignant progression to colon carcinoma in man; (5) some data suggest an effect of promoting agents on the invasiveness of human colon carcinomas; and (6) rationale intervention in colon carcinoma evolution may be possible since promotion at early stages is a reversible phenomenon.

We made human colon carcinoma development an experimental system by describing appropriate tissue culture techniques to place into primary culture normal colonic epithelial cells, early-stage premalignant colonic epithelial cells from familial polyposis and genetically high-risk non-polyposis patients (Friedman et al 1984a), and the more advanced premalignant cells composing adenomas (Friedman et al 1981). About 90% of all biopsies were culturable so no patient selection occurred, and the results were representative of the patient population. The epithelial cells migrated as a continuous sheet from partially digested explants. The cells were identified as epithelial by general morphology and the presence of characteristic epithelial subcellular structures including junctional complexes (tight junctions, gap junctions, and desmosomes in that order), interlocking adjacent cells, a brush border on the apical side facing the medium, the secretion of mucus, and the presence of goblet cells interspersed between the transporting cells within the epithelial sheets cultured from normal patients. The cells were also functionally epithelial, transporting water through the epithelial sheet and discharging it through the basal surface so that the accumulated fluid caused a bulging of the sheet. These fluid-filled domes were often observed.

The cells were studied without passage so the only selection was for viable cells able to migrate onto the surface of the dish. Migration is a normal characteristic of colonic epithelial cells which move up the colonic crypt as they differentiate and divide. The lymphocytes which make up the lamina propria were lost upon digestion of the colonic tissue, and the few fibroblasts which line the crypts did not migrate from the explants unless the epithelial cells which migrated first had died. The cellular sheets were monolayers of pure epithelial cells.

The tumor promoter TPA caused the release of the protease plasminogen activator from adenomas which contained dysplastic cells (23 of 24 cases) or a subpopulation of villous cells, and from each of 12 carcinomas (Friedman

1981; Friedman et al 1984b). This protease caused characteristic and easily detectable changes in the morphology of the secreting cells, causing cells to first elongate, then separate and form multicellular aggregates loosely attached to the petri dish. Adenoma epithelial cells grow in a tightly opposed flagstone pattern. Extensive membrane interdigitations, junctional complexes, and an extensive actin cable network unite adjacent cells into a tightly woven network. The cells also intercommunicate by a functional gap junction network as shown by the passage of a small molecular weight fluorescent dye to the cells adjacent to a dye-injected single cell within the adenoma monolayer. Carcinoma cells in primary culture do not compose a tightly organized network like adenoma cells. Individually dye-injected carcinoma cells transmit the fluorescent dye to, on the average, three adjacent cells (Friedman and Steinberg 1982) indicating a very small functional unit, probably daughter cells. The actin cable network characteristic of adenoma cells was completely lost in carcinoma cells, which displayed a few thin actin filaments in a halo around the cell's periphery (Friedman et al 1984c). TPA treatment of dysplastic adenoma cells and villous adenoma cells led to plasminogen-activator secretion. The secreted protease caused the morphological changes cited above and the adenoma cells then phenotypically resembled carcinoma cells.

What does this mean in biological terms for tumor development? The careful histopathology studies cited above from Morson's group have shown that colon carcinoma in man begins within a focus of dysplastic cells that in turn lies within an adenoma, most often a villous adenoma. These are the classes of adenoma cells which secrete plasminogen activator when promoted. All carcinomas tested also secreted this protease. When the carcinoma cell arises, probably by mutation of a preexisting adenoma cell, it is surrounded by adenoma cells which form a tightly interwoven cell network. We hypothesize that the carcinoma cell would be prevented from dividing by the contact inhibition of the surrounding adenoma cells if it and the surrounding cells did not secrete plasminogen activator when promoted (Fig. 1). The protease secretion is not envisaged as a one-step procedure, but a continuous process which slowly allows the carcinoma focus to grow within the adenoma.

The carcinoma cells must penetrate the adenoma to become invasive. The effect of the protease on adenoma cells is quite dramatic, and few adenoma cells after protease release remained viable for an extended period. In contrast, carcinoma cells from an established line, HT-29, continue to proliferate after repeated treatments with TPA. Co-cultivation of HT-29 carcinoma cells with adenoma cells has shown that the adenoma cells are invaded and destroyed by proteolysis while the carcinoma cells flourish (Friedman and Winawer, unpublished observation). These experiments, we believe, demonstrate how carcinoma cells overgrow and destroy the adenoma within which they arose. It may also explain why most carcinomas exhibit little, if any, adenomatous regions by the time they are resected. Therefore, absence of adenoma tissue from a carcinoma would not disprove the adenoma-carcinoma sequence. Our data predicts the destruction of most, if not all, of the host adenoma by the emerging carcinoma.

What of the remaining premalignant cell types? The remaining adenomas and the nontumor premalignant cells from patients genetically predisposed to develop colon cancer did not secrete a plasminogen-activator in response to TPA, but were stimulated to divide (Friedman 1981; Friedman et al 1984b; Friedman et al 1984a). These included all five tubular adenomas and epithelial cells from five of six familial polyposis patients. Promotion of these cells in vivo would lead to an increase in number of premalignant cells. The spontaneous mutation rate for a single, scorable trait in eukaryotic cells is estimated to be rather low, about one in a million cells. A mutagenic carcinogen which was not lethal in the body might increase that level 10 to 100 times. Increasing the number of premalignant cells would increase the likelihood that a mutation in a premalignant cell would be nonlethal and would lead to further tumor development.

Premalignant cells from nonpolyposis, high-risk patients did not respond to TPA by mitogenesis, demonstrating another difference between those cells and the ones characterizing familial polyposis patients. Normal epithelial cells from control subjects under the same conditions of in vitro culture also did not respond to TPA by mitogenesis (Friedman et al 1984a).

These data imply that all classes of human pre-malignant colonic epithelial cells, except the genetically high-risk, nonpolyposis cells, are promoted in vivo and when cultured, return to a ground state from which they can be promoted in vitro. Recently, data have been published which is consistent with our hypothesis; namely, that these premalignant cell types were promoted in vivo. Ornithine decarboxylase is an enzyme with elevated levels when cells are treated with a promoting agent; for example, mouse keratinocytes during skin carcino-genesis-promotion protocol (O'Brien 1975). Colonic mucosa from normal patients was found to have low levels of this enzyme, while mucosa from familial polyposis patients and adenomas exhibited higher levels. Dysplastic polyps exhibited the highest levels (Luk and Baylin 1984). There is a complete correlation between the tissues found with an elevated level of ornithine decarboxylase in vivo, and the tissues, which when cultured in vitro, respond to promoting agents.

Two compounds found in the colon may work together with promoting agents to increase the total mass of premalignant cells by selectively enhancing proliferation. Both epidermal growth factor and deoxycholic acid were found to stimulate the replication of premalignant cells from tubular adenomas, but not from villous adenomas (Friedman 1981: Friedman et al 1981; summarized in Table 1). Neither stimulated the release of plasminogen-activator from any cell type tested. Epidermal growth factor has a very strong structural homology to urgas-trone, a trophic hormone in the intestine. We include it in the media for normal and nontumor early-stage premalig-nant cells (Friedman 1984a). Lack of response to it at later stages in premalignant development may imply the secretion of a hormone by the cells themselves (autocrine response). Deoxycholic acid is a secondary bile acid found in the colon. Numerous animal studies have implicated it in colonic tumor development (references reviewed in Friedman 1981). We postulate that these agents increase the size of tubular adenomas to increase the likelihood of a mutation leading to more advanced, dysplastic adenomas.

The implication of tumor promotion in human colon carcinoma development offers some hope of developing rational therapies for this disease. Several compounds

Table 1: Effect of TAP, Deoxycholic acid (DOC), and Epidermal Growth Factor (EFG) on normal, Preneoplastic, and Malignant Human Colonic Epithelial Cells.

Cell Type	TPA	Response to EFG	DOC
Normal	No mitogenesis, 5 patients	Not tested (NT) but mitogenic	NT
Preneoplastic: Hereditary Syndromes a) Familial non-polyposis	No mitogenesis, 13 patients	NT	NT
b) Familial poly-posis	8-fold mitogenesis, 5 of 6 patients	NT	NT
Preneoplastic: Tubular adenoma	Mitogenesis averaging 71 ± 42%, 4 patients	Mitogenesis averaging 82 ± 33%, 3 patients	Mitogenesis averaging 93 ± 35%, 4 patients
Preneoplastic adenoma with villous and/or dysplastic cells	Plasminogen activator release, 16 of 18 patients	No plasminogen activator release no mitogenesis, 6 patients	No plasminogen activator release, no mitogenesis, 4 patients
Malignant	Plasminogen activator release, 12 patients	NT	NT

which block tumor promotion in vitro and in experimental
animals have been described. We are now in the process of
developing protocols to study certain of these compounds
on cultured human colonic premalignant cells.   In addition, tumor promoters need to be applied many times to
cause tumor development.   This is consistent with the
observed mitogenic effects of TPA, epidermal growth
factor, and deoxycholic acid on tubular adenoma cells. A
growth factor must either be present continually or
applied often to keep cells replicating at their maximal
rate.   Therefore, the disease might be arrested at a
premalignant state by interrupting the promotion of the
premalignant cells at this stage. Division of human colon
carinoma development into several distinct biological
stages suggests that both the type of tumor promoter and
its function varies with tumor development (Fig. 1, and
more detailed model in Friedman et al 1984b), and offers
several potential points to interrupt tumor evolution.

REFERENCES

Blumberg PM, Dunn JA, Jaken S, Jen AY, Leach KL, Skarkey
    NA, Yeh E (1984). Specific receptors for phorbol ester
    tumor promoters and their involvement in biological
    responses.   In Slaga TJ (ed):   "Mechanisms of Tumor
    Promotion", Vol 3, Boa Raton: CRC Press, p 1.
Friedman E (1981). Differential response of premalignant
    epithelial cell classes to phorbol ester tumor promoters
    and to deoxycholic acid. Cancer Res 41:4588.
Friedman EA, Steinberg ML (1982). Disrupted communication
    between late-stage premalignant human colonic epithelial
    cells by 12-0-tetradecanoylphorbol-13-acetate.   Cancer
    Res 42:5096.
Friedman EA, Higgins PJ, Lipkin M, Shinya H, Gelb AM
    (1981).   Tissue culture of human epithelial cells from
    benign colonic tumors. In Vitro 17:632.
Friedman E, Gillin S, Lipkin M (1984a). 12-0-Tetradecan-
    oylphorbol-13-acetate stimulation of DNA synthesis in
    cultured preneoplastic familial polyposis colonic
    epithelial cells but not in normal colonic epithelial
    cells. Cancer Res 44:4078.
Friedman E, Urmacher C, Winawer S (1984). A model for
    human colon carcinoma evolution based on the differen-
    tial response of cultured preneoplastic, premalignant,

and malignant cells to 12-0-tetradecanoylphorbol-13-ace-tate. Cancer Res 44:1568.

Friedman E, Verderame M, Winawer S, Pollack R (1984c). Actin cytoskeletal or ganization loss in the benign-to-malignant tumor transition in cultured human colonic epithelial cells. Cancer Res 44:3040.

Goerttler K. Loehrke H, Schweizer J, Hesse B (1979). Systemic two-stage carcinogenesis in the epithelium of the forestomach of mice using 7,12-dimethylbenz(a)anthrene as initiator and the phorbol ester 12-0-tetradecanoyl-phorbol-13-acetate as promoter. Cancer Res 39:1293.

Hennings H, Shores R, Wemk ML, Spangler EF, Tarone R, Yuspa SH (1983). Malignant conversion of mouse skin tumors is increased by tumor initiators and unaffected by tumor promoters. Nature 304:67.

Konishi F, Morson BC (1982). Pathology of colorectal adenomas: a colonoscopic survey. J Clin Pathol 35:830.

Lipkin M (1984). Method for binary classification and risk assessment of individuals with familial polyposis based on [^{3}H]TdR labeling of epithelial cells in colonic crypts. Cell Tissue Kinet 17:209.

Lipkin M, Blattner W, Fraumeni J, Lynch H, Deschner E, Winawer S (1983). Tritiated thymidine labeling distributions in the identification of hereditary predisposition to colon cancer. Cancer Res 43:1899.

Luk GD, Baylin SB (1984). Ornithine decarboxylase as a biologic marker in familial colonic polyposis. N Engl J Med 311:80.

Muto T, Bussey HJR, Morson BC (1975). The evolution of cancer of the colon and rectum. Cancer (Phila) 36:2251.

Nishizuka Y (1984). The role of protein kinase C in cell surface signal transduction and tumor promotion. Nature 308:693.

O'Brien TG, Simsimian RC, Boutwell RK (1975). Induction of the polyamine-biosynthetic enzymes in mouse epidermis by tumor-promoting agents. Cancer Res 35:1662.

Sugimura T (1982). Potent tumor promoters other than phorbol esters and their significance. Gann 73:499.

Carcinoma of the Large Bowel and Its Precursors, pages 187–202
© 1985 Alan R. Liss, Inc.

CELL KINETIC APPROACHES TO DEFINING PREMALIGNANT
CONDITIONS

Eleanor E. Deschner, Ph.D.
Head, Laboratory of Digestive Tract
  Carcinogenesis
Memorial Sloan-Kettering Cancer Center
New York, New York 10021

The presence of single or multiple adenomas in the
large bowel as well as the occurrence of inflammatory
bowel disease in this region pose a distinct risk for the
development of colon cancer. In both instances, the risk
increases with the duration of the condition. Thus, the
continued growth of the adenoma over a period of years or
the long-standing presence of ulcerative colitis increases
the malignant potential of the disease state.

What attributes do conditions involving adenomas and
ulcerative colitis share that predispose the colon to
cancer? It is this question which forms the basis of this
presentation. Certainly some comprehension of the preneoplastic alterations in the mucosa when either of these
disease states is present serves not only as a possible
approach to a greater understanding of the disease itself
and the biological events preceding cancer in general, but
may serve also as a basis for the development of better
treatment strategies.

Before discussing cell kinetics with regard to
adenomas and ulcerative colitis, it is necessary to
describe briefly the major techniques used to amass this
type of information. Most of the methods require that
tritiated thymidine (^{3}HTdR) be incorporated into the
proliferating epithelial cells and that the presence of
the radioactivity be recognized by autoradiography.
Colorectal biopsies incubated in nutrient medium to which
the isotope is added enable one to assess the labeling
index (L.I.) or percentage of cells engaged in DNA synthe-

sis as well as the distribution of these cells in the crypts.

Occasionally, [3]HTdR has been injected into a patient with limited life expectancy and biopsies taken at various intervals to follow the progress of a labeled cohort of cells. A labeled mitosis curve constructed with data collected over several days usually can provide estimates of the duration of the various phases of the cell cycle and the total cell cycle duration (T_c). With human tissue, however, often the only phases determined with some accuracy are the G_2 phase or the premitotic gap and the S phase or the DNA synthesis interval. The G_1 or presynthetic gap and T_c are frequently not obtained in man because of inadequate sampling after 24 hours. However, these phases have been obtained in rodents which have a shorter cell cycle duration.

Double labeling techniques using [3]HTdR and ^{14}C or a weak and a high dose of [3]HTdR and a known interval between their delivery have made it possible to estimate the duration of S phase and T_c in human biopsy material (Bleiberg et al 1970, 1972, 1977).

PRENEOPLASTIC CHANGES

A number of alterations in the proliferative behavior of colorectal epithelial cells have been recognized using an in vitro organ culture technique (Deschner 1982). Firstly, confirmation was obtained that in vitro labeling of animal and human tissue provided findings similar to that seen when labeling was carried out in vivo; in normal specimens cell proliferation was confined to the lower two-thirds of the crypts. However, in a number of disease states normal appearing mucosa showed [3]HTdR labeled cells extended to the luminal surface (Stage I defect) (Deschner et al 1963). This enlarged proliferative compartment (PC) was observed in patients with multiple or familial polyposis, patients with a history of colon cancer, individuals with an isolated polyp, asymptomatic relatives of familial polyposis patients, ulcerative colitis patients, and even some individuals in the general population.

A second abnormality was observed in the colorectal mucosa of patients with a history of cancer (Maskens and Deschner 1977). This proliferative defect was character- ized by a shift of the major zone of DNA synthesis from the lower third of the gland to the middle and upper portion of the crypts. This Stage II abnormality has been shown among patients with an isolated adenoma, individuals with some familial link to colon cancer as well as those with chronic ulcerative colitis. No control patients expressed the upward shift or Stage II defect.

This shift in proliferative activity was also seen in experimentally induced colon cancer at a time when focal areas of cellular atypism were evident in the middle and upper regions of the mucosa. The significance of the upward shift can be clarified by this DMH model which revealed crypts with a bulge or outpocket in the middle and upper wall after as few as three weekly injections of the carcinogen. Normally, new glands are formed from the base of the crypt as it undergoes fission, a process seen with frequency during postnatal growth. This enhanced proliferative activity in the middle and upper crypts (Stage II defect) apparently creates a cellular buildup which is released as an outpocket or lateral extension when the basement membrane stretches or enlarges to accommodate this growth.

An additional parameter (Stage III abnormality) has more recently been described by us as characterizing abnormal colonic epithelial cell behavior (Deschner and Maskens 1982). Crypts with extremely elevated labeling indices were identified in the mucosa of patients with a previous history of neoplasia. Only one of 13 control patients had crypt labeling indices greater than 15% whereas 17 of 26 cancer and polyp patients expressed this defect. When crypts in the patient population with tumors were separated into those with a low L.I. (<8%) and those with a high L.I. (>15%), it was noted that both types expressed Stage I and Stage II defects. However, glands with L.I. greater than 15% expressed both abnormalities more intensely suggesting that this third proliferative defect was indeed a later step in the development of neoplasia. Crypts with an extremely elevated L.I. have also been found in 1,2-dimethylhydrazine (DMH) treated CF$_1$ mice indicating that probably a similar developmental pattern leads to neoplasia in mice and in man.

What significance can be attributed to crypts with extremely elevated L.I.? Quite clearly, such glands have a selective advantage to express neoplastic potential earlier than crypts with a lower level of proliferative activity. Moreover when two or more of these hyperactive crypts appear in close proximity, it is likely that the tumor emerging will be large in a relatively short period of time. Moreover, this tumor would be characterized by two or more neoplastic clones with perhaps different karyotypes and different cell cycle times. Were the lesion to become malignant, the presence of two or more malignant stem cells would certainly complicate any chemotherapeutic program designed to eradicate the tumor. Perhaps at this point it is important to stress one obvious conclusion from all this, and that is the clearly independent nature of each single crypt. Each gland has its own indigenous set of controls governing all phases of proliferation and differentiation.

TUMOR GROWTH

Examination of tissue from familial polyposis patients and DMH treated mice has revealed that small adenomas are formed in the upper portion of the mucosa and the continued growth of the lesion and the development of new glands occurs by the downward invagination of the surface epithelium (Maskens 1979).

It is the upper luminal portion of the adenomatous glands which demonstrate the greatest degree of DNA synthesis activity. Thus the lesion grows by infolding and branching of the surface epithelium. The downward migration rate has been found to be 0.4 cell positions/ hour in adenomatous glands as opposed to a rate of 0.3 cell positions/hour in a luminal direction in the adjacent normal appearing mucosa (Lightdale et al 1982).

The continued infolding of the adenomatous epithelium increases the number of gland openings along the surface while the number of basal crypt formations remains stable. This results in the familiar convex upward trapezoid appearance of adenomas (Maskens 1979). It has been suggested by Maskens that the difference in morphology between adenomas and villous adenoma is attributable to the response of the mesenchymal elements. When the latter has great proliferative potential then outward folding of the adenomatous tissue occurs and a villous adenoma is formed. Whereas when the mesenchymal tissue has little proliferative potential, resistance is set up and infolding of the tumor tissue occurs and an adenoma results.

TUMOR KINETICS

Based on experimental colon tumor models it has been deduced that small tumors have a faster growth rate than larger tumors (Maskens 1978). Certainly microscopic adenomas in general have labeling indices higher than that of the normal appearing colonic mucosa and small lesions have higher L.I. than large tumors (Deschner and Raicht 1981; Maskens 1978). Moreover when a lesion arises, all the tumor cells have the ability to proliferate so that the growth fraction is 1.0 and the doubling time is close to the value of the cell cycle time. In general, the growth rate of the tumor then decays exponentially with increasing size of the tumor. Tumor growth then depends on the contribution of three factors - the mean cell cycle time of the tumor cells, the fraction of cells proliferating, and the degree of cell loss occurring due to necrosis or desquamation.

Table 1:

Kinetic Parameters of Human Adenomas

L.I. (%)		S Phase (hr)		Turnover Time (hrs)		
Normal	Adenoma	Normal	Adenoma	Normal	Adenoma	
9.3	13.0					Deschner and Raicht, 1981
35.1	33.5	10.1	9.5			Bleiberg, et al., 1977
10.4	22.9	8.3	7.4	80.0	32.7	Bleiberg, et al., 1972
	3.0		16.1		154.0	Lesher, et al., 1977
17.0		11.2		73.0		Bleiberg and Galand, 1976

Investigations into the fraction of tumor cells proliferating have been carried out on adenomas in both man and experimental models. A number of different approaches have been used to obtain the data and this may be a source of the variability in the reported results. In general, the L.I. observed in adenomas was higher than that of the normal appearing mucosa (Table 1). For example, adenomas in a familial polyposis patient had a mean L.I. of 13.0±6.9 (S.D.) compared with 9.3±1.6 for the flat mucosa (Deschner and Reicht 1981). While the range of L.I. for the normal mucosa of that patient was 6.2 to 10.5%, the range for the adenomas was 5.7 to 35.1%, over a six fold variability. There was also a wide spread of values among fragments of each biopsy, indicating differences from area to area in the same tumor. Small foci of dysplasia were found to show the highest levels of DNA synthesis, i.e., 35% of the cells in a focus of 77 epithelial cells were seen in S phase. A variety of values have been obtained by others using the in vitro labeling procedure for biopsy material (Bleiberg et al 1972, 1977). Bleiberg et al (1977) have noted that the L.I. of the flat normal appearing mucosa adjacent to polyps and tumors was three times higher than the value found in normal subjects. When tumor fragments are minced and single cells were incubated, L.I. on the order of 3% have been obtained (Lesher 1977) suggesting that loss of the proliferatively active cells may have occurred with a resultant selection of a slow growing cell line.

With regard to the cell cycle, alterations in some phases have been observed. An increased duration of G_2 has been noted in a villous adenoma compared with the adjacent flat mucosa. A duration of 15 hours was observed compared with 7-8 hours in the histologically normal tissue (Lipkin et al 1970). The S phase of the villous adenoma may also be longer. In vitro measurements in six polyps revealed S phases in the range of 6.2-13.5 hours with a mean of 9.5±1.1 compared with 10.1±0.5 hours in adjacent mucosa (Bleiberg et al 1977). Lesher had a range of 10-16 hours. In fact, S phase durations in colon adenocarcinomas appear to be prolonged - i.e., 15.2-22 hours vs. 9.0-16.2 hours in adjacent mucosa (Bleiberg and Galand 1976) suggesting a possible progressive prolongation of S phase to be associated with carcinogenesis. Such a theory was proposed almost 20 years ago by Hoffman and Post (1967).

As previously stated, estimated turnover times which assume all cells are proliferating and are homogeneously distributed in the cycle are equivalent to the cell cycle times (T_C). Under such conditions those values approximate the time necessary to double the number of cells provided cell loss does not occur. Such T_C for adjacent colonic mucosa ranged from 38 to 110 hours with a mean and S.E. of 73.0±6 hours (Bleiberg and Galand 1976). Lesher (1977), however, reported cell cycle times of 64.5 and 154 hours for villous adenomas and adenomatous polyps, respectively, with doubling times of the tumors calculated as 6.5 and 16.1 days.

EXPERIMENTALLY INDUCED ADNOMAS

The kinetics of chemically induced colonic neoplasms have also been examined (Table 2). Small focal areas of atypism induced by DMH had labeling indices which were higher than normal-appearing mucosa of the same animal. The tumor L.I. might be as much as 3 times that of the normal tissue. However, among lesions in the small animal, a 2-fold difference in the number of S phase cells was observed (Deschner 1974).

Table 2:

DMH Experimentally Induced Tumors

	L.I. (%)		Cell Cycle (hr)		S Phase (hr)		GF (%)		
	T	N	T	N	T	N	T	N	Reference
Adenomas	30	15							Wiebecke, 1973
Microadenomas	18	12					·		Deschner, 1975
Ademonas	18.2	8.9	23.2	23.2	6.1	9.9	60	33	Chang, 1979
Adenomas Subsurface	23.6	7.6	21	58.0	7.0	9.0			Sunter, 1980

T - Tumor

N - Normal or Normal Appearing

Some generalizations can be made from the several kinetic analyses carried out on DMH induced adenomas. Certainly when the tumors become visible they still reveal an increased level of cell proliferation; a level which was much higher than that of the normal appearing mucosa or control colonic mucosa. The L.I. of the adenoma is thought to approximate closely the L.I. of the proliferative compartmnt of colonic crypts, that is, approximately

21% (Chang et al 1979) suggesting that neoplastic cells originate from transformed stem cells. There appears to be some agreement that the duration of S phase is shortened in experimental adenomas and that G_1 and G_2 durations are lengthened, but a consistent pattern of altered cell kinetic parameters has not emerged, indicating a large degree of cellular and tumor heterogeneity even among neoplasms induced by the same carcinogen and in the same strain of rodent.

In general, it has been shown with DMH induced rat carcinomas that smaller tumors are more likely to have a higher L.I., a faster turnover time, and a shorter doubling time. With increasing tumor size, mean cell cycle times lengthen, and the growth fraction or fraction of cells which are proliferating decrease, and doubling times increase (Maskens 1978).

MODIFICATION OF CELL PROLIFERATION

Modification of cell proliferation in the colon has been demonstrated involving a variety of substances which are commonplace in the diet or related to diet - i.e.,

Table 3:

Effect of Dietary Agents on Cell Proliferation

in Control and Normal Appearing Carcinogen Treated

Colonic Mucosa of Rodents

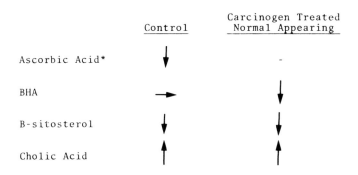

	Control	Carcinogen Treated Normal Appearing
Ascorbic Acid*	↓	-
BHA	→	↓
B-sitosterol	↓	↓
Cholic Acid	↑	↑

*Depresses proliferation in Familial Polyposis Colon

ascorbic acid (Deschner et al 1983a), B-sitosterol (Deschner et al 1982), butylated hydroxyanisol and bile acids (Deschner et al 1981) (Table 3). It is not known if these substances affect the growth of tumors but it is assumed that by either enhancing or depressing cell proliferation the number and growth of lesions will be affected (Deschner 1982).

Other endogenous factors such as hormones also influence colonic epithelial cell proliferation - i.e., the autonomic nervous system controls cell proliferation in the normal appearing crypts of the rat but does not appear to regulate tumor cell proliferation (Tutton and Barkla 1977). Histamine and very low doses of serotonin stimulate cell proliferation in DMH-induced colonic tumors (Tutton and Barkla 1978a and 1978b), whereas histamine H_2 receptor blockers such as cimetidine and inhibitors of serotonin synthesis retard cell proliferation. It has been theorized that the proximity of the sympathetic nerves as the source of noradrenaline at the base of the colonic crypt allows the localized stimulation of normal cell proliferation. Tumor cells however, lacking this close association to neural elements may adapt and acquire a sensitivity to another set of hormones; namely, the biogenic amines which can influence cell renewal and growth.

Yet another factor to be considered and one which appears to influence response to chemically induced tumor formation is the basic indigenous proliferative pattern characteristic of the biological subject. A correlation was shown to exist between mouse strains with variable susceptibility to DMH, and their characteristic colonic proliferative pattern (Deschner et al 1983c). CF_1 mice and the SWR strain of mice which demonstrate 100% DMH induced tumor incidence have a high L.I., a wide proliferative compartment, and a large percentage of proliferating cells in the middle third of the crypt. On the other hand, the AKR strain which is resistant to DMH tumor induction has a low L.I., a narrow PC, and a small percentage of DNA synthesizing cells in the middle third of the colonic glands. From these observations one may surmise that the higher population of S phase cells in the middle third of the CF_1 and SWR crypts influence the early transition and expansion of the PC to the upper third of the glands (Stage I abnormality) and the shift of the major zone of DNA synthesis to the middle and upper regions of the glands (Stage II abnormality). Suscepti- bility to these two proliferative defects within the CF_1 and SWR mucosa coupled with an already elevated L.I. allow DMH induced mutations to be stabilized, transmitted, and expressed in the future development of adenomas.

ULCERATIVE COLITIS

Several ulcerative colitis studies undertaken over the last 14 years have examined the tissue on a kinetic basis and each has provided a fresh insight into the character of the mucosa (Table 4). Bleiberg and his associates (1970) using a double label technique have demonstrated a high proliferating population in colitic mucosa compared with control patients, a relatively similar duration of S phase in both groups, and a short turnover time in the inflammatory bowel patients (31.2 hours vs. 90.0 hours). These general values have been confirmed by Biasco et al (1983). Eastwood and Trier (1973) demonstrated faster migration to the upper third of crypts in colitic mucosa, in addition to an enlarged proliferating population. This would explain the immature appearance of cells in the upper regions of the glands and the lack of differentiation noted there. Serafini and his group (1981) have shown that the proliferative character- istics of a mucosa with active ulcerative colitis is little different from a mucosa of a patient with ulcer- ative colitis in remission. Regardless of whether patients were in histological or sigmoidoscopic remission, or clinically active, proliferative indices were similar, L.I. = 15.5-18.8 range vs. 19.0±0.4, respectively. Thus, even in remission, epithelial cell proliferation was significantly higher than that seen in control patients. Moreover, extension of the proliferative compartment to the luminal surface was observed in both active colitics and colitics in remission.

Unfortunately, three studies do not confirm a high L.I. in the rectal mucosa of patients with ulcerative colitis in remission (Lehy 1983; Deschner 1983; Biasco 1983). No significant differences existed between the values reported by these investigators for patients in remission and that of control patients. Unlike Serafini, Biasco noted a decline in L.I. among colitics in remission and a more normal turnover time in the tissue. Moreover, a shift in the major zone of DNA synthesis from the lower third to the middle and upper third of the crypts was observed among the ulcerative colitis patients in these studies. Thirty-eight percent of colitis patients in Deschner's study, 17% in the ulcerative colitis group with an ileorectal anastomosis, and 14% of unoperated ulcerative colitics of Lehy's study and in 10 of 14 (71%) of Biasco's patients with inflammatory bowel disease for 10 years or longer exhibited this altered pattern of cell proliferation (Stage II abnormality). This loss of regulatory control over cell proliferation is apparently only one manifestation of a defect governing cell replication in these individuals. Certain patients with long-standing colitis have shown no depression in the level of DNA synthesis in the presence of phosphodiesterase inhibitors suggesting again a related breakdown in the mechanism controlling epithelial cell proliferation manifesting itself in a preneoplastic mucosa (Alpers et al 1980).

Table 4:

Ulcerative Colitis Studies - Rectal Mucosa

	S (hrs)	L.I. (%)	T_c (hrs)	Reference and Comment
Controls	7.9	9.5	90.0	Bleiberg, et al., 1970
UC	9.2	25.9	31.2	
Controls	-	4.8	-	Eastwood and Trier, 1973
UC	-	12.9	-	6hr incubation
Controls	-	13.1±0.5	-	Serafini, et al., 1981
UC Active	-	19.0±0.4	-	6hr incubation
UC Remission	-	15.9-17.9 (range)	-	
Controls	-	7.1±0.6	-	Lehy, et al., 1983
UC Remission	-	8.1±0.9	-	
IRA-UC Remission	-	8.9±0.5	-	
Controls	-	7.7±3.9	-	Deschner, et al., 1983
UC Remission	-	8.9±3.6	-	
Controls	7	9	80	Biasco, et al., 1983
UC Active	8	24	30	estimated values
UC Remission	7	11	75	

Clearly, markedly elevated levels of cell proliferation can be found in inflammatory bowel mucosa and there
are also remarkable variabilities between affected
individuals with the disease. Part of the discrepancies
in the data from different laboratories may be related to
the length of the incubation time employed. A 6-hour
incubation time cannot be considered pulse labeling and
runs the risk of allowing cells labeled at the S/G_2
interface to reach M/G_1 phase thereby artifactually
elevating the L.I. This is particularly disconcerting in
a disease entity such as ulcerative colitis which is
thought to have an already markedly shortened cell cycle
time.

We have been interested in establishing an animal
model for colitis and have investigated the use of
degraded carrageenan (Glaxo) as an inductive agent in CF_1
mice (Fath et al 1984). Ten percent carrageenan in the
drinking water induced bloody diarrhea, pericryptal
inflammation, and marked dilatation of the cecum and
ascending colon. While distorted crypt architecture,
inflammation of the lamina propria, and ulceration were
more pronounced in the proximal colon, they were also
present in the distal colon. Labeling indices were
significantly increased over control values in both
proximal (12.9±4.9 vs. 7.6±2.9) and distal colon (13.9±5.2
vs. 7.2±2.4) doubling the number of DNA synthesizing cells
per crypt column in both areas. Greater mucosal damage to
the proximal colon was reflected in the greater extension
of the proliferative compartment along the cryptal wall,
and only in the proximal colon did labeled cells appear in
the upper third or normally non-proliferative zone of the
glands. Administration of hydrocortisone and levamisole
concurrently with the 10% carrageenan reduced the severity
of the response although the proximal colon was less protected by both drugs than was the distal colon. Labeling
indices and labeled cells/column were consistantly lower
reflecting less damage and more protection in the distal
colon. This conclusion is reinforced when the effect of
hydrocortisone alone on colonic epithelial cell proliferation was examined. A significant depression in DNA
synthesis compared with control values was achieved only
in the distal colon (L.I. 4.0±1.0 vs. 7.2±2.4, p<0.01).
However, hydrocortisone in combination with 10%
carrageenan did not protect the distal colonic mucosa
uniformly. Rather, there remained crypt columns with

extremely large numbers of proliferating cells and these columns remained characterized by an extended proliferative compartment and high L.I.

Clarification of some of the inconsistencies previously related and confirmation of our animal model observations came about when we analyzed biopsies taken along the length of an operative specimen from an individual with long-standing ulcerative colitis. Not only was a greater than two-fold variability of L.I. shown among the biopsies (range 7.4-18.7%) but variability was further emphasized by the range of individual crypt L.I. which reach a maximum of 15.2-39.4% (unpublished observations). A large proportion of the crypts with elevated L.I. were further characterized by the presence of Stage I and II abnormalities. Thus, we see the focal nature of this disease and can only conclude that clinical remission is merely relative. The condition continues to be characterized by individual isolated crypts, many with abnormally distributed cells and many engaged in abnormally high levels of cell proliferation. Presumably these hyperactive crypts may undergo neoplastic transition in one of two ways. They appear capable of forming adenomatous tissue as well as capable of more direct malignant transformation. Obviously the continued presence of such crypts provides credibility to the persistent risk for malignancy which ulcerative colitis patients harbor within their mucosa.

In conclusion then, kinetic analyses indicate that adenomas and inflammatory bowel disease do indeed share a common proliferative defect and thereby a common risk for the development of colon cancer. Notably, it is the Stage III abnormality - namely, the continued uncontrolled level of cell proliferation - which confers on each of these tissues the increased opportunity for malignant transformation.

REFERENCES

Alpers DH, Philpott G, Grimme NL, Margolis DM (1980). Control of thymidine incorporation in mucosal explants from patients with chronic ulcerative colitis. Gastroenterology 78:470.

Biasco G, Miglioli M, Minarini A, Dalaiti A, DiFebo G, Gizzi G, and Barbara L (1983). Rectal cell renewal as biological marker of cancer risk in ulcerative colitis. In Sherlock P, Morson BC, Barbara L and Veronesi U (eds): "Precancerous Lesions of the Gastrointestinal Tract", New York: Raven Press, p 261.

Bleiberg H and Galand P (1976). In vitro autoradiographic determination of cell kinetic parameters inadenocarcinomas and adjacent healthy mucosa of the human colon and rectum. Cancer Res 36:325.

Bleiberg H, Mainguet P, and Galand P (1972). Cell renewal in familial polyposis: Comparison between polyps and adjacent healthy mucosa. Gastroenterology 63:240.

Bleiberg H, Mainguet P, Galand P, Chretien J and Dupont-Mairesse N (1970). Cell renewal in the human rectum. In vitro autoradiographic study on active ulcerative colitis. Gastroenterology 58:851.

Bleiberg H, Salhadin A and Galand P (1977). Cell cycle parameters in human colon. Comparison between primary and recurrent adenocarcinomas, benign polyps and adjacent unaffected mucosa. Cancer 39:1190.

Chang WWL, Mak KM and MacDonald PDM (1979). Cell population kinetics of 1,2-dimethylhydrazine-induced colonic neoplasms and their adjacent colonic mucosa in the mouse. Virchows Archiv (Cell Pathol) 30:349.

Deschner EE (1974). Experimentally induced cancer of the colon. Cancer 34:824.

Deschner EE (1982). Early proliferative changes in gastrointestinal neoplasia. Am J of Gastroenterology 77:207.

Deschner EE, Alcock N, Okamura T, DeCosse JJ and Sherlock P (1983a). Tissue concentrations and proliferative effects of massive doses of ascorbic acid in the mouse. Nutrition and Cancer 4:241.

Deschner EE, Cohen BI and Raicht RF (1981). Acute and chronic effect of dietary cholic acid on colonic epithelial cell proliferation. Digestion 21:290.

Deschner EE, Cohen BI and Raicht RF (1982). Kinetics of the protective effect of B-sitosterol against MNU induced colonic neoplasia. J Cancer Res and Clinical Oncology 103:49.

Deschner EE, Lewis CM and Lipkin M (1963). In vitro study of human epithelial cells I. Atypical zone of ^{3}H-thymidine incorporation in mucosa of multiple polyposis. J Clin Invest 42:1922.

Deschner EE, Long FC, Hakissian M and Herrmann SL (1983b). Differential susceptibility of AKR, $C_{57}BL/6J$ and CF_1 mice to 1,2-dimethylhydrazine-induced colonic tumor formation predicted by proliferative characteristics of colonic epithelial cells. J Natl Cancer Inst 70:279.

Deschner EE and Maskens AP (1982). Significance of the labeling index and labeling distribution as kinetic parameters in colorectal mucosa of cancer patients and DMH treated animals. Cancer 50:1136.

Deschner EE and Raicht RF (1981). Kinetic and morphologic alterations in the colon of a patient with multiple polyposis. Cancer 47:2440.

Deschner EE, Winawer SJ, Katz S, Katzka I, Kahn E (1983c). Proliferative defects in ulcerative colitis patients. Cancer Investigation 1:41.

Eastwood GL and Trier JS (1973). Epithelial cell renewal in cultured rectal biopsies in ulcerative colitis. Gastroenterology 64:383.

Fath RB, Deschner EE, Winawer SJ, Dworkin BM (1984). Degraded carrageenan-induced colitis in CF_1 mice - a clinical, histopathological and kinetic analysis. Digestion 29:197.

Hoffman J and Post J (1967). In vivo studies of DNA synthesis in human normal and tumor cells. Cancer Res 27:898.

Lehy T, Mignon M and Abitbol JL (1983). Epithelial cell proliferation in the rectal stump of patients with ileorectal anastomosis for ulcerative colitis. Gut 24:1048.

Lesher S. Schiffer LM and Phanse M (1977). Human colonic tumor cell kinetics: Potential for therapy. Cancer 40:2706.

Lightdale C, Lipkin M and Deschner EE (1982). In vivo measurements in familial polyposis: Kinetics and location of proliferating cells in colonic adenomas. Cancer Res 42:4280.

Lipkin M, Bell B, Stalder G and Troncale F (1970). The development of abnormalities of growth in colonic epithelial cells. In Burdette WJ (ed): "Carcinoma of the Colon and Antecedent Epithelium", Springfield: CC Thomas Publ., p 213.

Maskens AP (1978). Mathematical models of carcinogenesis and tumor growth in an experimental rat colon adenocarcinoma. In LipkinM and GoodRA (eds): "Gastrointestinal Tract Cancere", New York: Plenum Medical Book Co. p 361.

Maskens AP (1979). Histogenesis of adenomatous polyps in the human large intestine. Gastroenterology 77:1245.

Maskens AP and Deschner EE (1977). Tritiated thymidine incorporation into epithelial cells of normal-appearing colorectal mucosa of cancer patients. J Natl Cancer Inst 58:1221.

Serafini EP, Kirk AP and Chambers TJ (1981). Rate and pattern of epithelial cell proliferation in ulcerative colitis. Gut 22:648.

Sunter JP, Hull DL, Appleton DR and Watson AJ (1980). Cell proliferation of colonic neoplasma in dimethylhy-drazine-treated rats. Br J Cancer 42:95.

Tutton PJM and Barkla DH (1977). The influence of adreno-receptor activity on cell proliferation in colonic crypt epithelium and in colonic adenocarcinomata. Virchows Arch B 24:139.

Tutton PJM and Barkla DH (1978a). Stimulation of cell proliferation by histamine H_2 receptors in dimethyl-hydrazine-induced adenocarcinomata. Cell Biol Int Rep 2:199.

Tutton PJM and Barkla DH (1978b). The influence of sero-tonin on the mitotic rate in the colonic crypt epithelium and in colonic adenocarcinomata in rats. Clin Exp Pharmacol Physiol 5:91.

Wiebecke B, Krey U, Lohrs U and Eder M (1973). Morpho-logical and autoradiographical investigations on experi-mental carcinogenesis and polyp development in the intestinal tract of rats and mice. Virchows Arch (Pathol Anat) 360:179.

Carcinoma of the Large Bowel and Its Precursors, pages 203–215

COMPARATIVE HISTOGENESIS AND PATHOLOGY OF NATURALLY-OCCURRING HUMAN AND EXPERIMENTALLY INDUCED LARGE BOWEL CANCER IN THE RAT

Jerrold M. Ward, D.V.M., Ph.D., and
Masato Ohshima, M.D., Ph.D.
Tumor Pathology and Pathogenesis Section,
Laboratory of Comparative Carcinogenesis,
Division of Cancer Etiology, National Cancer
Institute, Frederick, Maryland 21701

Laboratory animals have been successfully utilized to develop experimental models of human disease in order to study and understand the etiology and pathogenesis of diseases in humans. Several chemicals have been used in rats to induce preneoplastic, precancerous, and neoplastic lesions of the large bowel, which resemble those observed in humans. This paper will review the model systems and the pathology of the induced large bowel tumors of rats in comparison with those of man.

MODEL SYSTEMS

A variety of experimental systems have been developed for studying large bowel cancer in rats. These include single or multiple injections of 1,2-dimethylhydrazine (DMH) (Fisher et al 1981; Madera et al 1983, Pozharisski 1975; Sunter et al 1978; Ward 1974), azoxymethane (AOM) (Shamsuddin, Trump 1981; Ward 1975; Ward et al 1973), methylazoxymethanol acetate, aminobiphenyls, recently feeding of tryptophan pyrolysis products (Takayama et al 1984), and intrarectal administration of N-nitroso-N-methylurea (NMU), or other nitroso compounds (Ward et al 1978; Ward et al 1977). Distribution of multiple neoplasms between specific regions of small and large intestines varies with dosage and differs from one experimental system to another. Also, specific types of tumors are induced by each chemical and treatment schedule. For example, DMH and AOM induce many polypoid tumors, invasive adenocarcinomas and metastatic mucinous adenocarcinomas in the colon (Pozharisski 1975; Ward 1974) while NMU induces primarily invasive tubular and cystic adenocarcinomas which do not metastasize (Ward et al 1978). High doses generally induce more tumors per rat, tumors with shorter latent period and an earlier mortality. For most model systems that involve injection, extracolonic tumors arise, as well, in various organs and may interfere with study of the large bowel tumors (Ward 1974). Intrarectal administration of a direct acting carcinogen, such as NMU eliminates this problem. These model systems have been utilized to study the modification of colon tumor development (tumor promotion or inhibition and carcinogenesis) by dietary constituents (fat, protein, and fiber), endogenous constituents (bile acids and bile salts) and exogenous factors (drugs and vitamins) (Autrup, Williams 1983; Zedeck 1978). Transplantable tumors have been developed for the study of therapeutic and biologic aspects of the colon tumors (Zedeck 1978).

HISTOGENESIS OF LARGE BOWEL TUMORS IN HUMANS

There is much epidemiological and histopathological evidence that clearly supports the concept that most colorectal adenocarcinomas not associated with ulcerative colitis or genetic disease evolve from preexisting tubular or villous adenomas (Corman et al 1975; Muto et al 1975) (Fig. 1) in spite of some disagreement to this hypothesis (Castleman, Krickstein 1962). An obvious association exists between prevalence of adenoma at autopsy and colon cancer incidence (Correa, Haenszel 1977); adenoma is more common in individuals with carcinomas (22% or 50%) than in those without carcinomas (12%) (Corman et al 1975; Ekelund 1974); and in long-term follow-up studies, individuals with adenomas have a significantly higher incidence of the development of colorectal carcinomas than those without adenomas (Corman et al 1975; Correa, Haenszel 1977; Muto et al 1975). The anatomic distribution of adenomas in clinical series frequently parallels that of carcinomas. Both are most common in the rectum and sigmoid (Appel 1982; Corman et al 1975; Ekelund 1974). Focal atypia and focal carcinomas are seen commonly in adenomas (in 5% to 40% of adenomas), while both findings are dependent on adenoma size, and remnants of adenoma are seen within 10% to 27% of the carcinomas (Corman et al 1975; Correa, Haenszel 1977; Lambert et al 1984; Lane et al 1978; Muto et al 1975). It must be noted, however, that apparent remnants of polyps may in fact represents adenomatous differentiation of carcinomas. A gradual increase in the average ages of patients parallels the advance of histologic atypism from adenomas with a low grade of invasive cancer (Kozuka et al 1975). It may take at least 5 years to 15 years for the adenoma-carcinoma sequence to evolve (Corman et al 1975; Correa, Haenszel 1977; Kozuka et al 1975; Muto et al 1975). There are similarities of histochemical and biological features of adenoma and carcinoma (Boland et al 1982; Isaacson 1982). Finally, aggressive removal of adenomas in populations reduces the incidence of colon cancer (Crespi et al 1984).

Adenoma thus has a distinct malignant potential. However, it is obvious that adenomas do not all have the same malignant potential. The prevalence of carcinoma from villous adenomas is eight times higher than that from 5 tubular adenomas (Muto et al 1975). The malignant potential of adenomas increases with the size and histopathologic grade of the adenomas. Although most pathologists agree that only a small percentage of carcinomas arise de novo, there are no detailed necropsy and serial section studies to prove this point. In addition, malignant changes can be seen in 1.3% of small adenomas under 1 cm (Muto et al 1975). Some of these lesions may be termed "mucosal dysplasia" or "carcinoma in situ". It cannot be denied that an unknown proportion of large bowel carcinomas arise de novo. We present the potential histogenesis of human colorectal adenocarcinoma as follows in Figure 1.

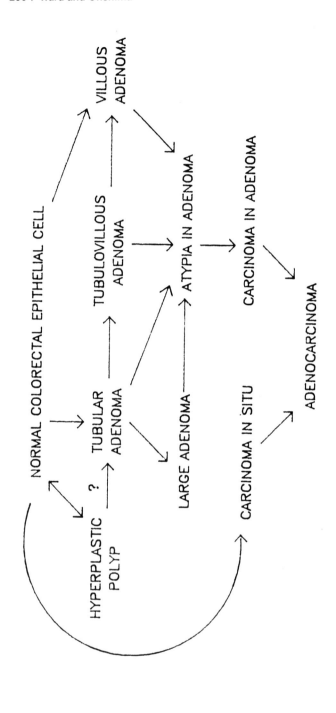

FIG. 1 — HYPOTHETICAL HISTOGENESIS OF NATURALLY—OCCURRING HUMAN LARGE BOWEL CANCER

HISTOGENESIS OF LARGE BOWEL TUMORS IN RATS

Each chemical carcinogen induces characteristic large bowel tumors with specific morphologic and biologic behavior. With most carcinogens, three types of tumors are induced (Pozharisski 1975; Pozharisski et al 1979; Ward 1974): (1) Polypoid neoplasms resembling human adenomas with moderate-to-severe degrees of atypia and dysplasia, growing as exophytic tumors (Figs. 2, 3), and with common stalk invasion (Fig. 4). Unlike human adenomas displaying focal carcinoma which invades the stalk, polypoid tumors invade the stalk without evidence of a new focal malignant change in the tumor; (2) tubular adenocarcinomas, arising de novo from flat colonic epithelium growing as endophytic tumors (Figs. 5, 6); and (3) mucinous adenocarcinomas which arise de novo and metastasize in more than 50% of the rats (Ward 1974). The histogenetic scheme is given in Fig. 7.

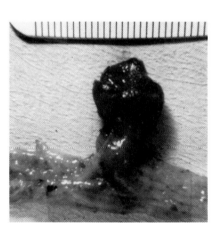 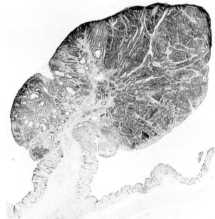

Fig 2 - Gross appearance of rat colonic polyp

Fig 3 - Rat colonic adenoma without stalk invasion.

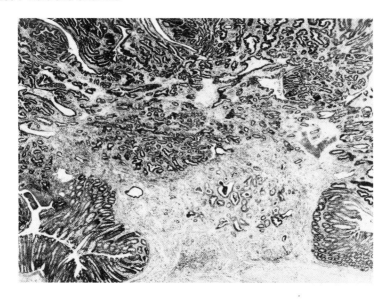

Fig. 4 - Invasion of stalk by large polypois tumor.

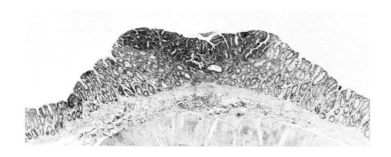

Fig 5 - Intraepithelial carcinoma (superficial cancer) in
rat colon.

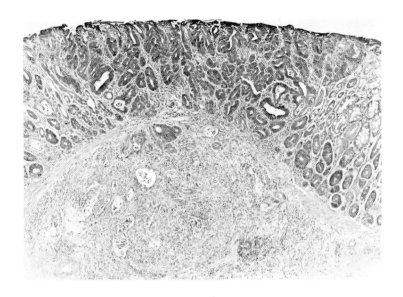

Fig. 6 - Small colonic carcinoma arising <u>in situ</u> and invading into submucosa.

Polypoid neoplasms have been variously claimed to be
adenomas, adenomas in all stages of progressive malignancy
(Madera et al 1983; Sumter et al 1978) and polypoid adenocarcinomas of low grade malignancy (Maskens, Dujardin-
Loits 1981; Ward 1975). These tumors arise in flat epithelium <u>de novo</u> and have characteristics of moderate-to-
severe dysplasia from their time of origin (Kikkawa 1974;
Maskens, Dujardi-Loits 1981; Lindstrom 1978; Pozharrisski
1975; Maskens 1981; Shamsuddin et al 1981; Sunter et al
1978; Ward 1974; Ward 1975; Ward et al 1973; Wiebecke et
al 1973). These early neoplastic lesions have been termed
superficial cancer when intraepithelial in location and
carcinoma in situ (Pozharisski 1975) when the lamina propria is involved (Fig. 8).

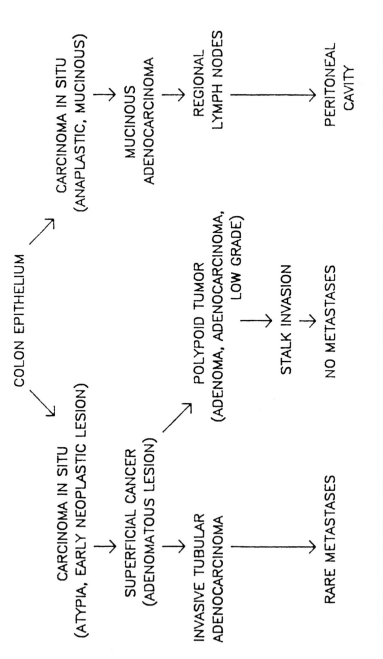

FIG. 7 – HISTOGENESIS AND NATURAL HISTORY OF CHEMICALLY–INDUCED RAT LARGE BOWEL CANCER SHOWING SYNONYMS FOR THE SAME LESIONS BY VARIOUS AUTHORS

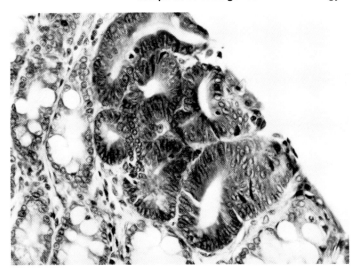

Fig. 8 - The earliest neooplastic lesion in rat colon
induced by carcinogens. It has been diagnosed as
carcinoma in situ, focal atypia and dysplasia and
adenomatous hyperplasia.

These early lesions of polypoid tumors are usually
indistinguishable from those that appear to progress to
small invasive tubular adenocarcinomas, which invade
progressively through the muscularis mucosae, submucosa,
and tunica muscularis. There is a direct association
between diameter of the tubular adenocarcinoma and depth
of invasion of the colon wall (Ward et al 1978). In contrast, the tumors which develop into polypoid tumors grow
into the colon lumen but have severe-to-moderate diffuse
atypia usually indistinguishable from that on the surface
of invasive adenocarcinomas. Almost from the beginning,
the tumors which grow as polypoid adenomas (Figures 3, 4)
have a disrupted muscularis mucosae and invade their
stalks to various degrees (Ward 1975; Ward et al 1973).
The degree of invasion may be more severe in larger tumors
(Figure 4) although this process originates in small
tumors.

Invasive tubular adenocarcinomas and stalk invasion
of polypoid tumors are characterized by similar scirrhous
and inflammatory reactions (Madera et al 1983; Ward 1974).
Occasionally, invasive tumor cells are better differenti-

ated (have less atypia, hyperchromatism and more cyto-plasm) than do tumor cells on the luminal surface of the same tumor. Although polypoid tumors frequently have stalk invasion, they rarely show invasion into the tunica muscularis and essentially never metastasize.

EFFECT OF CARCINOGEN, CARCINOGEN DOSE, AND TREATMENT SCHEDULE ON POLYPOID TUMOR MALIGNANCY

There has been no demonstrable effect of carcinogen dose or multiple treatment schedule on pathology of the induced tumors including invasion of the stalk of polypoid tumors and ultimate metastasis. In some published reports, as a percentage of total colon tumors, more polypoid tumors are found with some carcinogens than with others. In a few reports, low doses of carcinogens induce more invasive tubular and mucinous adenocarcinomas than polypoid tumors (Ward 1975) while at least one report shows more polypoid tumors at low doses (Ward et al 1978), perhaps similar to the human situation in low colon cancer incidence areas.

RAT COLON CANCER MODELS AND THE NATURAL HISTORY OF HUMAN LARGE BOWEL ADENOMAS AND CANCER

A study of the pathology of chemically induced colon tumors in rats provides much evidence for understanding the genesis of human large bowel tumors. Many of the rat tumors arise de novo from flat epithelium (Maskens, Dujar-din-Loits 1981; Pozharisski 1975; Ward 1974), which occurs in human ulcerative colitis and perhaps rarely in other people. Although foci of invasive carcinoma arise within polypoid tumors of rats, the more common and highly inva-sive and metastatic tumors arise de novo in rats while they apparently arise within adenomas in humans. Thus a quantitative difference is observed between rats and humans. The rat model offers a method to study the dose and other effects of carcinogens on the natural history of colon tumors. Further study of the rat models may aid in understanding the etiology and genesis of human polyps and carcinomas arising within polyps.

REFERENCES

Appel MF (1982). Distribution of malignant polyps in the colon. Dis. Colon Rectum 25:427.

Autrup H, Williams GM (1983). Experimental colon carcinogenesis. Boca Raton: CRC Press, pp. 320.

Boland CR, Montgomery CK, Kim YS (1982). A cancer-associated mucin alteration in benign colonic polyps. Gastroenterology 82:664.

Castleman B, Krickstein HI (1962). Do adenomatous polyps of the colon become malignant? NEJM 267:469-475.

Corman ML, Veidenheimer MC, Coller JA (1975). Recent thoughts on the development of colorectal cancer. Medical Clinics of North America 59:347.

Correa P, Haenszel W (1977). The epidemiology of large-bowel cancer. Adv Cancer Res 26:1.

Crespi M, Weissman GS, Gilbertsen VA, Winawer SJ, Sherlock PS (1984). The role of protosigmoidoscopy in screening for colorectal neoplasia. Ca-A Cancer J Clin 34:158.

Ekelund G (1974). On colorectal polyps and carcinoma with special reference to their interrelationship. Malmo, Sweden. pp. 63.

Isaacson P (1982). Immunoperoxidase study of the secretory immunoglobulinsystem in colonic neoplasia. J Clin Pathol 34:14.

Kikkawa N (1974). Experimental studies on polypogenesis and carcinogenesis of the large intestine. Med J Osaka Univ 24:293.

Kozuka S, Nogaki M, Ozeki T, Masumori S (1975). Premalignancy of the muscosal polyp in the large intestine; II. Estimation of the periods required for malignant transformation of mucosal polyp. Dis Colon Rectum 18:494.

Lambert R, Sobin LH, Waye JD, Stalder GA (1984). The management of patients with colorectal adenomas. Ca-A Cancer J Clin 34:167.

Lane N, Fenoglio CM, Kaye GI, Pascal RR (1978). Defining the precursor tissue of ordinary large bowel carcinoma implications for cancer prevention. In Lipkin M, Good RA (eds): "Gastrointestinal Tract Cancer", New York: Plenum, pp 295.

Lindstrom CG (1978). Experimental colorectal tumours in the rat. Acta Pathol Microbiol Scand A, Suppl 268, pp 75.

Madera J, Harte P, Deasy J, Ross D, Lahey S, Steele Jr. G (1983). Evidence for an adenoma-carcinoma sequence in dimethylhydrazine-induced neoplasms of rat intestinal epithelium. Am J Pathol 110:230.

Maskens AP (1981). Confirmation of the two-stage nature of chemical carcinogenesis in the rat colon adenocarcinoma model. Cancer Res 41:1240.

Maskens AP, Dujardin-Loits RM (1981). Experimental adenomas and carcinomas of the large intestine behave as distinct entities. Most carcinomas arise de novo in flat mucosa. Cancer 47:81.

Muto T, Bussey HJ, Morson BD (1975). The evolution of cancer of the colon and rectum. Cancer 36:2251.

Pozharisski KM (1975). Morphology and morphogenesis of experimental epithelial tumors on the intestine. J Natl Cancer Inst 54:1115.

Pozharisski KM, Kilhachev AJ, Klimasherski VF, Shaposhnikov JD (1979). Experimental intestinal cancer research with special reference to human pathology. Adv Cancer Res 30:165.

Shamsuddin AKM, Trump BF (1981). Colon epithelium. II. In vivo studies of colon carcinogenesis. Light microscopic, histochemical, and ultrastructural studies of histogenesis of azosymethane-induced colon carcinomas in Fischer 344 rats. J Natl Cancer Inst 66:389.

Sunter JP, Appleton DR, Wright NA, Watson AJ (1978). Pathological features of the colonic tumours induced in rats by the administration of 1,2-dimethylhydrazine. Virchows Arch Cell Path 29:211.

Takayama S, Masuda M, Mogami M, Ohgaki H, Sato S, Sugimura T (1984). Induction of cancers in the intestine, liver and various other organs of rats by feed mutagens from glutamic and pyrolystae. Gann 75:207.

Ward JM (1975). Dose response to a single injection of azoxymethane in rats. Vet Pathol 12:165.

Ward JM (1974). Morphogenesis of chemically induced neoplasms of the colon and small intestine in rats. Lab Invest 30:505.

Ward JM, Sporn MB, Wenk ML, Smith JM, Feeser D, Dean RJ (1978). Dose response to intrarectal administration of N-methyl-N-nitrosourea and histopathologic evaluation of the effect of two retinoids on colon lesions induced in rats. J Natl Cancer Inst 60:1489.

Ward JM, Rice JM, Roller PP, Wend ML (1977). Natural history of intestinal neoplasms induced in rats by a single injection of methyl (acetoxymethyl) nitrosamine. Cancer Res 37:3046.

Ward JM, Yamamoto RS, Brown CA (1973). Pathology of intestinal neoplasms and other lesions in rats exposed to azoxymethane. J Natl Cancer Inst 51:1029.

Wiebecke B, Krey U, Lohrs U, Eder M (1973). Morphological and autoadiographical investigations on experimental carcinogenesis and polyp development in the intestinal tract of rats and mice. Virchows Arch Ab A Path Anat 360:179.

Zedeck MS (1978). Experimental colon carcinogenesis. In Lipkin M, Good RA (eds): "Gastrointestinal Tract Cancer", New York: Plenum, pp. 343.

Carcinoma of the Large Bowel and Its Precursors, pages 217–235
© **1985 Alan R. Liss, Inc.**

THE MODE OF FORMATION AND PROGRESSION OF CHEMICALLY INDUCED COLONIC CARCINOMA

William W. L. Chang, M.D., Ph.D.
Department of Pathology
West Virginia University School of Medicine
  and University Hospital
Morgantown, West Virginia 26506

The proper understanding of the histogenesis of colon cancer is crucial to its prevention. However, carcinogenesis is a focal and sequential process and the detection of an early neoplastic lesion has created a great deal of technical difficulty.

To overcome some of these difficulties, we have turned to an animal model, since a fairly reliable induction of colorectal carcinoma has been achieved in rodents (Druckrey 1970; LaMont and O'Gorman 1978; Pozharisski et al 1979; Chang 1984). In rats, chemically induced colonic neoplasms are mostly short-stalked and isolated, being scattered throughout the large intestine, but in mice, they are sessile and numerous, being located mostly in the distal colon (Wiebecke et al 1973). Hence, the mouse appears to be a better model for investigating the early phase of colonic tumorigenesis, particularly in relation to the renewal behavior of the epithelial cells in the colonic crypt. Meanwhile, we have employed the autoradiographs of Epon-embedded sections of the distal colon of mice given tritiated thymidine, frequently of semi-serial or serial sections. Such preparations have given us a better way of determining the cellular changes by the cytology and proliferative activity of the cells concerned. With these improvements, we have attempted to answer specifically the following questions:

(1) Since there is evidence that a colonic epithelial neoplasm arises from a single crypt (Bussey 1975: Chang 1978), what is the mode of formation of

a colonic neoplasm in a single crypt, particularly in relation to renewal behavior of epithelial cells in the crypt?

(2) Following the formation of an early colonic neoplastic lesion, is the tumor growth process a multistep one? If so, what are the regulatory mechanisms of each step?

(3) There are currently two different views on the origin of colon carcinoma: adenoma-carcinoma sequence and de novo origin. Can the histogenetic studies of the early stages of colonic carcinogenesis shed some light on this controversy?

In this chapter, I have attempted to answer the above questions by summarizing our data on the mode of formation and progression of symmetrical 1,2-dimethylhydrazine (DMH) induced colonic epithelial neoplasms in mice. Much of this work has been presented previously (Chang 1978, 1982; Chang et al 1979).

MODE OF FORMATION OF NEOPLASM IN COLONIC CRYPT

In mammals, the crypt of Lieberkühn constitutes a structural unit of the colonic epithelium in which the epithelial cells are constantly proliferating in the lower and middle portion, migrate upwards along the crypt wall to differentiate concomitantly, and then migrate out of the crypt to the surface epithelium where they are extruded (Messier, Leblond 1960; Chang, Leblond 1971a). In the distal colon of the mouse, the crypt contains three lineages of epithelial cells: (1) columnar, or vacuolated-columnar cells, (2) goblet mucous cells, and (3) enteroendocrine (argentaffin) cells. There is evidence that these three cell lineages originate in a common stem cell or stem cells situated at the crypt base (Chang and Leblond 1971a,b). In the major cell line, the vacuolated-columnar cell line, vacuolated cells, (also known as deep crypt, non-goblet mucous cells (Spicer 1965; Wetzel et al 1966; Thomopoulos et al 1983), constitute the proliferative compartment and columnar cells the non-proliferative compartment. In the mucous cell line, there is a gradual transition in the morphology of cells by accumulating more mucus to form a goblet shape as proliferative mucous cells become non-proliferative ones (Figure 1).

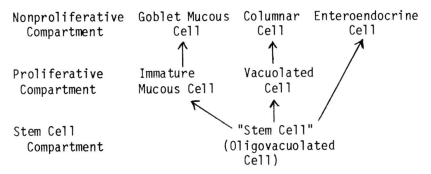

Cell Lineages in the Crypt of the
Murine Distal Colon

Figure 1: Cell lineages in the crypt of the distal colon of the mouse.

Under physiological conditions, most crypts in adult animals are in a steady state in terms of production, migration, and loss of epithelial cells. There are five critical events in the life of epithelial cells to maintain the steady state of the crypt: (1) stem cells to maintain the stem cell population; (2) differentiation into the three cell lineages from stem cells; (3) changeover of differentiating epithelial cells from the proliferative to non-proliferative status; (4) migration of non-proliferative, differentiated epithelial cells out of the crypt to the surface epithelium; and (5) extrusion of "worn-out", terminally differentiated epithelial cells from the surface epithelium (Chang 1982, 1984). The regulatory mechanisms of each of these events are still poorly understood. When neoplastic changes occur in a particular crypt, drastic changes are observed in relation to these events.

It should be emphasized that the crypt is a dynamic structure. Its size, shape, and cellularity depend on the rate of proliferation, migration, and extrusion of the epithelial cells. During the growth period of mammals, the rate of production of epithelial cells in the crypt exceeds the rate of migration of these cells out of the crypt. As a result, the number of epithelial cells in the crypt increases; this is often associated with an increase in the girth of the crypt starting at the crypt base where the putative stem cell compartment exists. With continuous increase in epithelial cell production, an epithelial budding originates at the crypt base, increases in height and forms a septum to divide a crypt into two (Figure 2). During this dichotomic process, the upward growth of the epithelial septum carries connective tissue elements and is accompanied by differentiation of epithelial cells from the proliferative to the non-proliferative status.

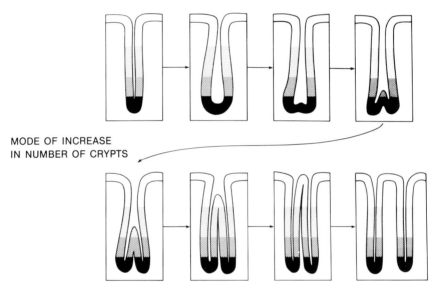

MODE OF INCREASE
IN NUMBER OF CRYPTS

Figure 2: The mode of crypt division during growth. The black, two differently dotted, and white areas of the crypt designate four generations of crypt epithelial cells based on the work of Chang and Nadler (1975). The epithelial budding occurs at the crypt base (stem cell compartment) and the growth of the epithelial septum is associated with epithelial cell proliferation and differentiation similar to the normal epithelial cell renewal. (Reproduced from Virchows Arch. Cell Pathol. with permission).

Administration of DMH to susceptible strains of mice, including CF-1 mice, causes degeneration of many epithelial cells in the proliferative compartment of the crypt as an acute cytotoxic manifestation (Lohrs et al 1969; Chang 1981; Sunter et al 1981; Wargovich et al 1983) and induces hyperplasia of the colonic crypt and hypertrophy of colonic mucosa when the carcinogen is given repeatedly (Wiebecke et al 1973; Thurnherr et al 1973; Kikkawa 1974; Chang 1978). In the hyperplastic crypts, the number of epithelial cells lining the crypt column increases as a result of an increase in cell proliferation. There is also an expansion of the proliferative compartment of the crypt, but the distribution of the tritiated thymidine-labeled cells follows the slow cut-off model of Cairnie et al (1965). This indicates that the changeover from the proliferative cells to the non-proliferative cells takes place in the upper part of the hyperplastic crypt as in the normal intestinal crypt. The hyperplastic crypts, therefore, represent reactive changes to the chronic administration of carcinogen and they are not the direct precursor of colonic neoplasms, although partial defects in the differentiation of epithelial cells are frequently observed (Chang 1978).

The changes specific for colonic tumorigenesis commence with carcinogen-induced neoplastic transformation of epithelial cells in the colonic crypt. However, isolated, neoplastically transformed cells can hardly be identified with certainty even in plastic embedded colonic sections, although there is some evidence that neoplastic transformation of epithelial cells following DMH treatment occurs in the proliferative compartment of the crypt. When a crypt is partly or entirely replaced by a group of cytologically atypical cells, such identification becomes possible. This type of crypt is called atypical or dysplastic (Chang 1982) (Figure 3). These dysplastic crypts commonly appear by nine weeks after initiation of DMH treatment in the mouse model.

Our studies have shown that there are two possible modes of crypt repopulation by atypical cells to form a dysplastic crypt (Chang 1982). In one mode, a given crypt appears to be repopulated from the base upwards by atypical cells and their clones subsequent to repopulation of the crypt base by neoplastically transformed cells. Such

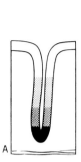 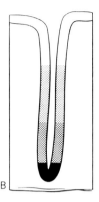 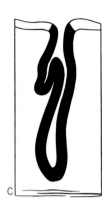

Figure 3: Normal colonic crypt (A) is compared to hyperplastic crypt (B) and dysplastic crypt (C) seen about 9-12 weeks after initiation of weekly injection of DMH. The black, two differently dotted and white areas represent four generations of epithelial cells as explained in Figure 2. Dysplastic crypts are repopulated by atypical cells resembling to some extent the putative stem cells at the cryptal base.

crypts are characterized by increased diameter, smooth contour and dilated lumen in the lower half and some irregularity and tortuosity with some evagination of the lining epithelium in the upper half. Mucous cell differentiation may occur but is usually defective, and mucous cells formed tend to be prematurely extruded from the epithelial lining into the crypt lumen (Chang 1978). At or around the mouth of the crypt, a sharp border between the repopulating atypical cells and remaining non-neoplastic epithelial cells can be seen. Apparently due to a block of migration of proliferating atypical cells at the crypt mouth, atypical cells accumulate in the upper part of the crypt to form an early neoplastic lesion.

In the other mode, a small outpocketing pouch consisting of atypical cells is formed somewhere in the proliferative compartment of a crypt, probably being associated with a defective basement membrane. Concomitant with the growth of the pouch, the mouth of the pouch appears to move upwards. Eventually the upper portion of the mother crypt is replaced by atypical cells, where an early neoplastic lesion is formed.

These findings are schematically summarized in Figure 4. It is probable that many isolated, neoplastically transformed cells occur anywhere in the proliferative compartment of the crypt following carcinogen treatment, but the majority of these cells migrate in cohort with the adjacent non-neoplastic epithelial cells along the crypt wall to the surface epithelium where they are extruded.

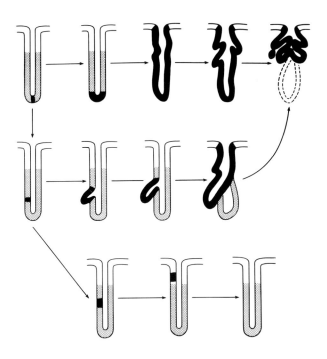

Figure 4: The possible modes of repopulation of a crypt by neoplastically transformed cells leading to the formation of an early neoplastic lesion (two upper rows). A majority of isolated, neoplastically transformed cells seem to migrate along the crypt wall with non-neoplastic epithelial cells and are extruded from the surface epithelium (bottom row). The dotted area shows the proliferative compartment of the crypt, whereas the black area represents the area occupied by neoplastically transformed cells. (Reproduced from Virchows Arch. Cell Pathol. with permission).

Only when they replace the crypt base or form an outpocketing pouch, do they appear to succeed in repopulating the given crypt to form a dysplastic crypt, probably within several days. In the dysplastic crypt, atypical cells seem to migrate upwards, but apparently due to a block at or around the crypt mouth, these cells accumulate in the upper portion of the crypt. The latter causes stagnation of epithelial cell migration and leads to cystic degeneration and disappearance of the lower portion of the mother crypt.

MODE OF PROGRESSION OF COLONIC CARCINOMA

An early neoplastic lesion that is derived from a single dysplastic crypt and formed in the upper part of the mucosa is composed of a rather homogeneous population of atypical cells with frequent tritiated thymidine-labeled cells and mitoses. The cytology of atypical cells varies more among the lesions than within the lesion. The neoplastic lesions exhibit varying degrees of dysplastic changes: some being adenomatous, some moderately dysplastic, and others adenocarcinomatous. At the outset, the lesion is a relatively simple glandular structure but becomes increasingly complex with growth. Although dysplastic crypts may contain a few scattered partially differentiated mucous cells, the early neoplastic lesions are generally devoid of mucous cells. These early neoplastic lesions can be observed by nine weeks after the initiation of DMH treatment, but they are more frequently observed by 11 to 12 weeks.

The neoplastic glandular lesions formed in the upper part of the mucosa grow, expand and progress in various directions with time and at varied rates, depending on their intrinsic growth activity and interaction with the microenvironment. With continuous increase in the proliferative activity, the neoplastic glandular structures elongate and become tortuous and their epithelial lining becomes evaginated when the basement membrane is intact. Serial sections reveal that many neoplastic glands have an opening on the surface, some having a wide opening. At the mouth of the opening, the border between the atypical cells in the neoplastic gland and the non-neoplastic cells in the surface epithelium is observed. Meanwhile an epithelial budding occurs at or near the basal portion of the neoplastic gland usually located at the mid-portion of the mucosa, and grows to form a papillary projection, which increases in height to reach the level of the surface epithelium. If such a septum is a complete one, the neoplastic gland is divided into two, somewhat similar to the dichotomy process seen in normal intestinal crypts. However, when the epithelial septum is incomplete, a villous structure is formed. In contrast to the dichotomy process of normal crypts, epithelial septa formed in the neoplastic glands are not accompanied by full differentiation of the constituent epithelial cells. These observations explain why varying proportions of villous structures may be present in many colonic epithelial neoplasms. On the other hand, the neoplastic glandular structures may manifest greater variations in their morphology if there is an associated defect in their basement membrane. The epithelial lining may invaginate into the surrounding lamina propria and form an outpocketing pouch, and even their constituent neoplastic cells may invade into the lamina propria to manifest early malignant behavior. The alterations of the basement membrane occur frequently in various carcinomas (Barsky et al 1983; Ingber et al 1981; Liotta et al 1983), including colonic carcinoma (Burtin et al 1982). They are secondary to a defective formation of basement membrane by neoplastic cells and/or to elaboration of type IV collagenase by neoplastic cells (Liotta et al 1977, 1979). The penetration of the basement membrane by neoplastic cells appears to be a breakdown of an initial host defense barrier against the neoplasm, probably indicating an earliest phase of malignant behavior. This may be observed while the neoplasm is still limited to the mucosa. In conjunction with cytological alterations, such a neoplasm may be designated as intramucosal carcinoma. Usually there is no stromal reaction to such penetration.

Since each neoplastic lesion differs from every other in its cytology, proliferative activity, and integrity of the basement membrane as well as the relationship to its microenvironment, it is very difficult to predict its biological behavior on the basis of its morphology. It should be emphasized that there is a whole spectrum of manifestations by the neoplastic lesions and thus a simple classification of these lesions into benign or malignant ones creates a great deal of difficulty at the early stages of neoplastic development.

A neoplasm originating in a single dysplastic crypt is likely to be of monoclonal origin. During the growth, however, two or more adjacent neoplastic lesions may coalesce and thus a larger colonic neoplasm may be of multiclonal origin.

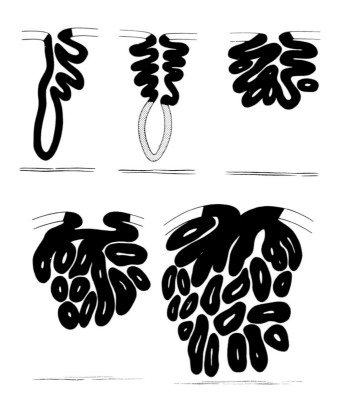

Figure 5: The mode of growth and expansion of colonic neoplasm within the mucosa following the formation of an early neoplastic lesion in the upper part of the mucosa from a dysplastic crypt.

Probably due to some variations in the proliferative activity within the neoplastic lesions and also to interaction with the microenvironment, the neoplasm may grow in various directions at varied rates (Figure 5) and may progress to a sessile polypoid form or a discoid form.

The most important factor in determining the biological behavior of the neoplasm is its downward progression. The deeper the neoplasm advances downward in the mucosa, the more aggressive it tends to be.

By 25 to 26 weeks after the initiation of DMH treatment, some neoplasms grow and progress downward to occupy the entire thickness of the mucosa. Meanwhile, the leading downward edges of the neoplastic glands appear to move in a serpentine fashion, creep along the muscularis mucosae, and penetrate this muscular layer at what seems to be a weak spot, setting the stage for a sequence of invasive behavior characteristic of malignant neoplasms. Apparently the muscularis mucosae constitutes a second host defense barrier against the progression of colonic neoplasms.

As soon as the muscularis mucosae is pierced by neoplastic glands, there is rearrangement of fibroblasts in the submucosa. The infiltrating neoplastic glands are usually concentrically surrounded by fibroblasts and collagen fibers. There is an increased production of collagen and proteoglycans of the extracellular matrix of the submucosa. In human colonic carcinomas, there is a 20-fold increase in the concentration of chondroitin 4-sulfate and 6-sulfate as compared to the normal colonic mucosa (Iozzo et al 1982). It has also been demonstrated that a hyaluronic acid-binding glycoprotein known as hyaluronectin (Delpech et al 1979) is present in the connective tissue surrounding the malignant glands (Burtin et al 1980). Therefore, the invasion of colonic wall beyond the muscularis mucosae appears to involve changes in both collagen and proteoglycan contents of the extracellular matrix. Apparently such connective tissue reaction constitutes a third host defense barrier to respond to neoplastic progression.

As the neoplasm invades further into the colonic wall, there is loosening, dissolution, and distintegration of the muscularis externa. Morphologically, the breakdown of this fourth host defense barrier seems to be due to the release of some lytic factors by the neoplastic cells and/or host cells surrounding the neoplastic glands. Neoplasms are known to produce some diffusible substances such as tumor angiogenesis factor (Folkman 1974), collagenase (Dresden et al 1972; Liotta et al 1981) dipeptidase (Sylven and Bois 1960), and proteinase (Poole et al 1978) among others. Host cells such as fibroblasts and leukocytes surrounding the invasive neoplastic glands produce a proteinase, cathepsin B, which appears to play a major role as activator of extracellular collagenase in the neoplasm (Graf et al 1981). Hence, various lytic factors released by the neoplasm and/or host cells seem to be closely related to the invasive behavior of the neoplasm.

Eventually the neoplasm may invade the vascular or lymphatic vessels and metastasize. However, metastasis is very infrequent in animal models, and the mode of metastasis of these chemically induced neoplasms has not been analyzed in detail.

Our morphological studies indicate that colonic carcinogenesis is a multistep process and is associated with successive breakdown of the host defense barriers. Four distinct but continuous steps which we have demonstrated include:

(1) repopulation of a given crypt by atypical epithelial cells to form a dysplastic crypt, which have either originated at the crypt base or occurred as an outpocketing pouch in the proliferative compartment of the crypt;

(2) formation of an early neoplastic lesion in the upper part of the dysplastic crypt;

(3) growth, expansion, and progression of neoplastic lesions in different directions by various mechanisms; and

(4) penetration of muscularis mucosae and the deeper portions of the colonic wall by the neoplasm to manifest apparent malignant behavior with successive breakdown of the host defense barriers in the colonic wall.

ADEMOMA-CARCINOMA SEQUENCE VERSUS DE NOVO ORIGIN OF COLONIC CARCINOMA

There has been a great deal of controversy regarding the origin of colonic carcinoma. Currently, pathologists are of the general opinion that most colonic carcinomas arise from preexisting adenomas (Fenoglio, Lane 1974; Muto et al 1975; Morson 1976), but some pathologists believe in the de novo formation of colonic carcinomas as they have found examples of small adenocarcinoma without adenomatous components. Even with the introduction of animal models for colonic carcinoma, such controversy still persists. In contrast to human colonic carcinoma, many investigators (Ward 1974; Pozharisski 1975; Maskens, Dujardin-Loits 1981) have claimed the de novo origin of chemically induced colonic carcinoma in experimental animals. Other investigators (Madera et al 1983) favor the adenoma-carcinoma sequence because they have demonstrated residual adenomatous components in colonic carcinomas induced in rats.

Animal experiments have shown that both adenomas and adenocarcinomas can be produced by the same carcinogens (Spjut and Spratt 1965; Thurnherr et al 1973; Wiebecke et al 1973; Pozharisski 1975). This indicates that they share a common etiologic factor. Since a large amount of carcinogen is administered in animal models within a short period, the induction and progression of colonic neoplasms are generally rapid without demonstrable adenomatous component within induced carcinoma, leading many investigators to conclude the de novo origin of colonic carcinoma. In man, small but undetermined amounts of unidentified carcinogens may be absorbed at irregular intervals, and thus colonic tumorigenesis seems to be a relatively slow process, and may be arrested for indeterminate periods at different stages of development and progression secondary to environmental factors including diet. Hence, human colonic neoplasms show more diversity in morphology and biological behavior than murine neoplasms, and it is not surprising to observe numerous examples of the adenoma-carcinoma sequence.

Based on our analysis of the histogenesis of colonic neoplasms, both adenomas and adenocarcinomas are more or less the end stages of evolution of neoplastically transformed cells. In the early stage, neoplastically transformed cells (morphologically identifiable as atypical cells) repopulate the given crypt to form a dysplastic crypt, from which an early neoplastic lesion is formed in the upper portion of the colonic mucosa. Each of these lesions is somewhat different, and there is a spectrum of cytological alterations, proliferative activity, and glandular organization of constituent atypical cells in these early neoplastic lesions. At this stage, it is very difficult to determine if the lesion is benign or malignant. In other words, the mode of formation of benign and malignant colonic neoplasms does not appear to differ significantly in the early stages of neoplastic development. However, the eventual mode of evolution of these lesions appears to differ, probably depending on the degree of their proliferative activity, cytological alterations, and interaction with the microenvironment.

In certain instances, the dysplastic crypt or the early neoplastic lesion subsequently formed are repopulated by severely dysplastic cells and go on to evolve into adenocarcinoma more or less similar to the mode described by the proponents of the de novo origin of colonic carcinoma. Most of these lesions tend to be small and discoid in appearance with the involvement of the entire thickness of the mucosa with subsequent invasion of the submucosa and the deeper portion of the colonic wall.

In many instances, neoplastically transformed cells repopulate the given crypt and form an early neoplastic lesion in the upper part of the mucosa, which gradually grows and expands to form a polypoid adenomatous lesion. Many of these polypoid neoplasms tend to expand and to progress downward slowly, and remain as benign neoplasms over a long period of time. However, at any stage of evolution to adenomas, neoplastic lesions may develop dysplastic foci, which may evolve into malignant neoplasms depending on microenvironmental factors. Varying proportions of adenomatous components may thus be observed in various stages of evolution of adenocarcinoma, supporting the adenoma-carcinoma sequence.

Therefore, it appears that both views on the origin of colonic carcinoma can be integrated in the scheme of the evolution of neoplastically transformed cells to adenomas and adenocarcinomas as presented in Figure 6.

In conclusion, the histogenesis of colonic neoplasms is a complex process, which can be dissected into various steps. The understanding of the mechanisms of each step of colonic tumorigenesis is essential for the prevention of colon cancer.

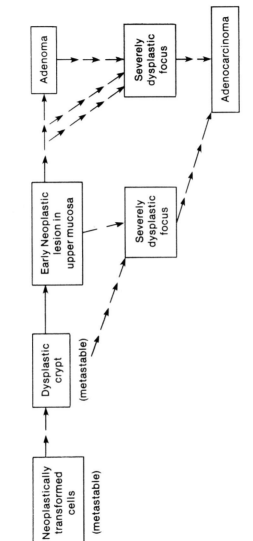

Figure 6: The mode of evolution of neoplastically transformed cells to adenoma and adenocarcinoma. (Reproduced from a supplement to the Scand. J. Gastroenterol. [in press] with permission).

REFERENCES

Barsky SH, Siegal GP, Jannotta F, Liotta LA (1983). Loss of basement membrane components by invasive tumors but not by their benign counterparts. Lab Invest 49:140-147.

Burtin P, Chavanel G, Foidart JM, Martin E (1982). Antigens of the basement membrane and the peritumoral stroma in human colonic adenocarcinomas: an immunofluorescence study. Int J Cancer 30:13-20.

Bussey HJR (1975). Familial Polyposis Coli. Baltimore: Johns Hopkins University Press.

Cairnie AB, Lamerton LJ, Steel GG (1965). Cell proliferation studies in the intestinal epithelium of the rat. II. Theoretical aspect. Exp Cell Res 39:539-553.

Chang WWL (1978). Histogenesis of symmetrical 1,2-dimethylhydrazine-induced neoplasms of the colon in the mouse. J Natl Cancer Inst 60:1405-1418.

Chang WWL (1981). Degenerative behavior of epithelial cells in the colonic crypt of the mouse following administration of colonic carcinogen, 1,2-dimethylhydrazine. Cancer Lett 13:111-118.

Chang WWL (1982). Morphological basis of multistep process in experimental colonic carcinogenesis. Virchows Arch Cell Pathol 41:17-37.

Chang WWL (1984). Histogenesis of colon cancer in experimental animals. Scand J Gastroenterol Supplement. (in press).

Chang WWL, Leblond CP (1971a). Renewal of the epithelium in the descending colon of the mouse. I. Presence of three cell populations: vacuolated-columnar, mucous and argentaffin. Am J Anat 131:73-100.

Chang WWL, Leblond CP (1971b). A unitarian theory of the three populations of epithelial cells in the mouse large intestine. Anat Rec 169:293.

Chang WWL, Mak KM, Macdonald PDM (1979). Cell population kinetics of 1,2-dimethylhydrazine-induced colonic neoplasms and their adjacent colonic mucosa in the mouse. Virchows Arch Cell Pathol 30:349-361.

Chang WWL, Nadler NJ (1975). Renewal of the epithelium in the descending colon of the mouse. IV. Cell population kinetics of vaduolated-columnar and mucous cells. Am J Anat 144:39-56.

Delpech B, Delpech A, Girard N (1979). An antigen associated with mesenchyme in human tumors that cross-reacts with brain glycoprotein. Br J Cancer 40:123-133.

Dresden MH, Heilman SA, Schmidt JD (1972). Collagenolytic enzymes in human neoplasms. Cancer Res 32:993-996.

Druckrey H (1970). Production of colonic carcinomas by 1,2-dialkylhydrazines and azoxyalkanes. In Carcinoma of the Colon and Antecedent Epithelium (Burdette, W.J. ed.), Springfield, Ill.: C.C. Thomas, pp 267-279.

Fenoglio CM, Lane N (1974). The anatomical precursor of colorectal carcinoma. Cancer 34:819-823.

Folkman J (1974). Tumor angiogenesis factor. Cancer Res 34:2109-2113.

Graf M, Baica A, Strauli P (1981). Histochemical localization of cathepsin B at the invasion front of the rabbit V2 carcinoma. Lab Invest 45:587-596.

Ingber DE, Madri JA, Jamieson JD (1981). Role of basal lamina in neoplastic disorganization of tissue architecture. Proc Natl Acad Sci, USA 78:3901-3905.

Iozzo RV, Bolender RP, Wight TN (1982). Proteoglycan changes in the intercellular matrix of human colon carcinoma. An integrated biochemical and stereologic analysis. Lab Invest 47:124-138.

Kikkawa N (1974). Experimental studies on polypogenesis and carcinogenesis of the large intestine. Med J Osaka Univ 24:293-314.

LaMont JT, O'Gorman TA (1978). Experimental colon cancer. Gastroenterology 75:1157-1169.

Liotta LA, Kleinerman J, Ctanzaro P, Rynbrandt D (1977). Degradation of basement membrane by murine tumor cells. J Natl Cancer Inst 58:1427-1431.

Liotta LA, Lanzer WL, Garbisa S (1981). Identification of a type V collagenolytic enzyme. Biochem Biophys Res Commun 98:184-190.

Liotta LA, Rao CN, Barsky SH (1983). Tumor invasion and the extracellular matrix. Lab Invest 49:636-649.

Liotta LA, Shigeto A, Robey PG, Martin GR (1979). Preferential digestion of basement membrane collagen by an enzyme derived from metastatic murine tumor. Proc Natl Acad Sci USA 76:2268-2272.

Lohrs U, Wiebecke B, Eder M (1969). Morphologische und autoradiographische Untersuchung der Darmschleimhautveranderungen nach einmaliger Injektion von 1,2-dimethylhydrazin. Z Ges Exp Med 151:297-307.

Madara JL, Harte P, Deasy J, Ross D, Lahey S, Steele G Jr (1983). Evidence for an adenoma-carcinoma sequence in dimethylhydrazine-induced neoplasms of rat intestinal epithelium. Am J Pathol 110:230-235.

Maskens AP, Dujardin-Loits RM (1981). Experimental adenomas and carcinomas of the large intestine behave as distinct entities: most carcinomas arise de novo in flat mucosa. Cancer 48:81-89.

Messier B, Leblond CP (1960). Cell proliferation and migration as revealed by radioautography after injection of thymidine-H^3 into male rats and mice. Am J Anat 106:247-285.

Morson BC (1976). Genesis of colorectal cancer. Clin Gastroenterol 5:505-542.

Muto T, Bussey HJR, Morson BC (1975). The evolution of cancer of the colon and rectum. Cancer 36:2251-2270.

Poole AR, Tiltman KJ, Recklies AD, Stoker TAM (1978). Differences in secretion of the proteinase, cathepsin B, at the edges of human breast carcinomas and fibroadenomas. Nature 273:545-547.

Pozharisski KM (1975). Morphology and morphogenesis of experimental epithelial tumors of the intestine. J Natl Cancer Inst 54:1115-1135.

Pozharisski KM, Likhachev AJ, Klimashevski VF, Shaposhnikov JD (1979). Experimental intestinal cancer research with special reference to human pathology. Adv Cancer Res 30:165-237.

Spicer SS (1965). Diamine methods for differentiating mucosubstances histochemically. J Histochem Cytochem 13:211-234.

Spjut HJ, Spratt JS Jr (1965). Endemic and morphologic similarities existing between spontaneous colonic neoplasms in man and 3:2'-dimethyl-4-aminobiphenyl induced colonic neoplasms in rats. Ann Surg 161:309-324.

Sunter JP, Appleton DR, Watson AJ (1981). Acute changes occurring in the intestinal mucosae of rats given a single injection of 1,2-dimethylhydrazine. Virchows Arch Cell Pathol 36:47-57.

Sylvan B, Bois I (1960). Protein content and enzymatic assay of interstitial fluid from some normal tissues and transplanted mouse tumors. Cancer Res. 20:831-836.

Thomopoulos GN, Schulte BA, Spicer SS (1983). Light and electron microscopic cytochemistry of glycoconjugates in the rectosigmoid colonic epithelium of the mouse and rat. Am J Anat 168:239-256.

Thurnherr N, Deschner EE, Stonehill EH, Lipkin M (1973). Induction of adenocarcinoms of the colon in mice by weekly injections of 1,2-dimethylhydrazine. Cancer Res 33:940-945.

Ward JM (1974). Morphogenesis of chemically induced neo-plasms of the colon and small intestine in rats. Lab Invest 30:505-513.

Wargovich MJ, Medline A, Bruce WR (1983). Early histo-pathologic events to evolution of colon cancer in C57BL/6 and CF-1 mice treated with 1,2-dimethylhydra-zine. J Natl Cancer Inst 71:125-131.

Wetzel MG, Wetzel BK, Spicer SS (1966). Ultrastructural localization of acid mucosubstances in the mouse colon with iron-containing stains. J Cell Biol 30:299-315.

Wiebecke B, Krey U, Lohrs U, Eder M (1973). Morphological and autoradiographical investigations on experimental carcinogenesis and polyp development in the intestinal tract of rats and mice. Virchows Arch Pathol Anat 360:179-193.

Carcinoma of the Large Bowel and Its Precursors, pages 237–245
© **1985 Alan R. Liss, Inc.**

THE CARRAGEENAN MODEL FOR EXPERIMENTAL ULCERATIVE COLITIS

Andrew B. Onderdonk, Ph.D.

Infectious Diseases Research Laboratory
Tufts University School of Veterinary Medicine
Boston, Massachusetts 02130

The increased incidence of intestinal cancer among individuals with inflammatory bowel disease (IBD) is a well recognized phenomenon. Of interest to investigators working in the area of intestinal cancer is whether animal model systems for IBD are also models for intestinal cancer. Among the inflammatory bowel diseases which affect humans, ulcerative colitis has received considerable attention due to the proximity of lesions to a large resident microflora and the proven ability of this microflora to produce chemical irritants.

Ulcerative colitis in humans is a large bowel disease characterized by periodic exacerbations and remissions, certain histopathologic markers and an uncertain etiology. Despite exhaustive clinical studies and analysis from virtually every scientific perspective, the etiology of this disease has remained elusive. An important part of the ongoing studies of this disease are the use of animal model systems which duplicate, to some extent, the clinical manifestations of the disease in humans. Attempts to define a useful animal model system generally can be classified into several groups (Table 1). It is interesting to note that each of these model systems have certain similarities to the disease process as noted in humans, despite the obvious anatomic differences, method of induction, and species studies. Unfortunately, the somewhat predictable response of the colon to toxic insult by a variety of agents makes it difficult to identify a model system which truly represents the same disease process described in humans.

TABLE 1

ANIMAL MODEL SYSTEMS FOR ULCERATIVE COLITIS

NATURAL	INDUCED	ALTERED HOST
canine	carrageenan	immune
porcine	infectious	vascular
rodent	microflora/metabolites	
equine		
marmoset		

Despite these drawbacks, our understanding of the experimental inflammatory process may yield useful information relevant to the human disease. It is the purpose of this report to review the carrageenan model for ulcerative colitis, the potential etiologic mechanisms associated with this model, and to discuss the potential role of the guinea pig as a chronic IBD model for use in large bowel cancer research.

CARRAGEENAN MODEL:

In 1969, Watt and Marcus first described the effect of degraded carrageenan on guinea pigs when a solution of this material served as the sole source of oral fluids for these animals. These investigators noted that animals given carrageenan uniformly developed cecal and large bowel ulcerations within 30 days after initiation of carrageenan treatment (Marcus and Watt 1969). Histopathologic evaluation of animals revealed crypt abscesses, polymorphonuclear cells in the lamina propria, increased cellularity, epithelial thinning, and obvious ulcerations. These observations have since been confirmed in the guinea pig by several investigators (Watt, Marcus 1973; van der Waaij et al 1974; Onderdonk et al 1977; Grosso et al 1973). The inducing agent used for these experiments, carrageenan, is an extract of red seaweeds such as Eucheuma spinosum and Chondrus crispus with gel characteristics in the native state similar to agar. Carrageenan is a sulfated polysaccharide of anhydro galactose and galactose with varying sulfate content and irregular branching (Watt, Marcus 1969: Mottet 1972). Acid hydrolysis of the native material results in the formation of fragments of smaller molecular weight with gel characteristics different than the native material. It is the low molecular weight (30,000 mw) material which appears to have activity in the guinea pig, while higher molecular weight material is commonly used as a suspending and thickening agent in foods and confections. Although reports have been published which indicate that large intestinal ulcerations occur in other animal species, the most consistent reports of carrageenan activity in an animal system are for the guinea pig.

Recent studies utilizing the guinea pig-carrageenan model have focused on the potential involvement of the intestinal microflora in the disease process (Onderdonk 1984). The model employed for these studies includes administration of a 5% w/v solution of degraded carrageenan to male, Hartley strain guinea pigs weighing 300-400 grams. Within 14-21 days of beginning administration of degraded carrageenan, the guinea pig's large bowel begins to exhibit histologic evidence of disease. The first changes noted consist of infiltration of the lamina propria and mucosal epithelium with polymorphonuclear and mononuclear cells, followed by epithelial thinning, loss of crypts and hyperemia. Microscopic ulcerations are generally seen first in the cecum by the 14-21st day and gradually become more severe during continued carrageenan administration until the animals become moribund and die. At the time of death the entire colon is often involved with gross and microscopic ulcerations. The cause of death in many cases is due to Gram negative sepsis coupled to extensive mucosal degeneration in the large bowel. It has been shown by Onderdonk (Onderdonk et al 1978) that administration of aminoglycosides to these animals decreases the mortality in this model system, but does not reduce the numbers of ulcerations. Additional studies of the intestinal tissues from carrageenan-treated animals reveal loss of haustral folds, mucosal granularity, crypt abscesses, lymphocytic infiltration, capillary congestion, pseudopolyps, and strictures. These findings have been confirmed and reviewed by a number of investigators over a period of 15 years.

ROLE OF THE INTESTINAL MICROFLORA IN THE CARRAGEENAN MODEL

Early studies with the guinea pig model were designed to determine whether indigenous bacteria of the intestinal microflora played any role in the experimental disease process. The strategy used for these studies employed quantitative enumeration and identification of the principal members of the microflora during carrageenan administration. It was shown that the total numbers of Gram negative facultative and obligate anaerobic species increased during carrageenan treatment, but no single species emerged as the dominant member of an altered microflora (Onderdonk et al 1977; Onderdonk and Bartlett 1979). Subsequent studies have utilized selective antimicrobial probes to determine whether supression of one or more components of the intestinal microflora altered the outcome of the experimental disease process. Gentamicin was selected to supress the coliform population, because of its activity against the facultative Gram negative organisms and because it lacked activity against obligate anaerobes. Metronidazole was selected because of its excellent and very specific activity against obligate anaerobes. Antimicrobial agents were given for three days prior to and concomitant with 5% degraded carrageenan for a total of 21 days. At the end of the experimental period, surviving animals were sacrificed and tissues removed for evaluation. It was found that the group receiving gentamicin had a reduced mortality versus the untreated carrageenan control, while the group receiving metronidazole showed a decrease in the number of animals with cecal ulcerations (Onderdonk et al 1978). These data suggested that coliforms were responsible for the mortality detected in this model, but did not alter the number of animals with ulcerations. On the other hand, metronidazole reduced ulcerations but not mortality. It was concluded that bacteria, probably obligate anaerobes, played some role in the development of the experimentally induced lesions. Additional experiments were designed to determine whether metronidazole was capable of decreasing the numbers of cecal ulcerations once ulcerations had already been formed. It was shown that delaying metronidazole therapy until the 14-21st day of carrageenan treatment did not result in any decrease in the numbers of animals with cecal ulcerations as compared to an untreated carrageenan control group. These data suggested that the role of bacteria in this model system occurred early and that the events which initiated the disease process might be different than those which sustained the later histologic abnormalities (Onderdonk et al 1978).

In an effort to better understand the role of bacteria in this model system, germfree guinea pigs were used as a method to determine whether carrageenan per se was responsible for the cecal ulcerations noted in conventional animals. Germfree guinea pigs were maintained on carrageenan for periods of 6 months prior to sacrifice yet none of these animals revealed cecal or large bowel abnormalities at necropsy. Additional experiments were performed in which animals were selectively associated with either a microflora obtained from gnotobiotic mice or from conventional guinea pigs. Subsequent treatment of these animals with carrageenan resulted in cecal ulcerations in the animals associated with the flora from conventional guinea pigs, but not in the group associated with the microflora from gnotobiotic mice (Onderdonk et al 1981). These data indicated that bacteria were required for cecal ulcerations to occur. More importantly, the results suggested that there was some specificity to the bacterial microflora required since the flora derived from mice was not capable of contributing to cecal ulcerations.

A further definition of the microflora required for cecal ulcerations in this model was attempted by isolating pools of 10-11 organisms to be used to associate germfree guinea pigs; 5% carrageenan solutions were provided as the sole source of oral fluids. Two of the derived pools of bacteria were capable of contributing to cecal ulcerations when guinea pigs were placed on carrageenan. Phenotypic characterization of these pools revealed one species common to both, Bacteroides vulgatus (Onderdonk et al 1981). Subsequent experiments utilizing this species by itself for mono-association of guinea pigs resulted in the identification of B. vulgatus as one bacterial species capable of contributing to cecal ulceration in the absence of other microflora. The identification of a single species capable of contributing to carrageenan-induced colitis invited obvious speculation about the mechanism by which B. vulgatus participated in the histopathologic changes associated with this model.

ROLE OF BACTEROIDES VULGATUS IN THE EXPERIMENTAL MODEL:

The identification of a single microbial species which contributed to cecal ulceration provided an opportunity to determine the specific manner in which microbes might contribute to this experimental model. Studies were performed in which B. vulgatus was fed to animals in the presence and absence of carrageenan to determine whether some factor produced by this species was responsible for enhancing the ulcerations noted with carrageenan treatment. None of the animals fed B. vulgatus alone developed cecal ulcerations or evidence of intestinal ulcerations. Although some of the animals given carrageenan exhibited a more intense inflammatory response, no significant difference in the number of intensity of lesions could be shown when compared to recipients of carrageenan alone. Additional experiments were conducted using B. vulgatus to immunize animals prior to carrageenan treatment and feeding of viable organisms. It was found that animals immunized with B. vulgatus prior to carrageenan treatment and feeding of the viable homologous strain developed more severe ulcerations at a more rapid rate than the corresponding non-immune groups (Onderdonk et al 1983). An identical experiment performed with B. fragilis, a phenotypically similar organism, did not reveal any increased cecal ulcerations. These data suggest that there is some specificity to the immune enhancement noted with B. vulgatus.

An inflammatory response following immunization with and monoassociation with B. vulgatus has also been noted in germfree mice (Onderdonk et al 1983). These animals developed a mononuclear infiltrate, pronounced epithelial thinning, and revealed polymorphonuclear cells within the lamina propria following association, but no ulcerations were detected. The ability of B. vulgatus to provoke an inflammatory response in two animal species suggests that this organism may possess some unique factor(s) which contribute to a local immune response in the intestine. This hypothesis as a mechanism by which ulcerative colitis occurs in humans is not unique (Shorter et al 1970a; Shorter et al 1970b; Shorter et al 1971; Watson 1969; Kirsner and Palmer 1954). There are, however, several alternative hypotheses regarding the role of carrageenan in the guinea pig model and in the human disease.

POSSIBLE ROLE OF CARRAGEENAN IN HUMAN ULCERATIVE COLITIS AND COLON CANCER:

The potential role of carrageenan in human ulcerative colitis and colon cancer is of keen interest to a variety of investigators. The higher molecular weight carrageenans are common additives to a number of foods in most "western" diets (Gorback 1971). In addition, these seaweed extracts serve as a staple in the diets of certain populations. Interestingly, there does not appear to be any correlation between consumption of carrageenans and human IBD or colon cancer.

There are several reports in the literature which indicate that administration of 10% degraded carrageenan solutions to rodents results in a higher incidence of colon cancer after several months of treatment (Oohashi et al 1981; Oohashi et al 1979; Wakabayashi et al 1978; Fabian et al 1973). These reports do not include the use of germfree animals; therefore, separation of the role of carrageenan per se and the role of an altered intestinal microflora or degradation products from carrageenan cannot be evaluated. That carrageenan administration results in a chronic inflammation of the large intestine of many animal species containing an intestinal microflora is well established. Whether carrageenan alone is a primary cause of colon cancer in animals or humans remains to be proven. It is clear that the guinea pig model provides an interesting system in which the progression of a chronic inflammatory process can be followed. Additional study will be required to determine whether colon cancer in this model, separate from that expected with any chronic IBD, resulted from carrageenan use.

REFERENCES

Fabian RJ, Abraham R, Coulston F and Goldberg L (1973). Carrageenan-induced squamous metaplasia of the rectal mucosa in the rat. Gastroenterology 65:265-276.
Gorbach SL (1971). Intestinal microflora. Gastroenterology 60:1110-1129.
Grosso P, Sharratt M, Carpanini FMB. Studies on carrageenan and large bowel ulceration in mammals. 11:555-564.
Kirsner JB and Palmer WL (1954). Ulcerative colitis: Considerations of its etiology and treatment. JAMA, 155:341-346.
Marcus R and Watt J (1969). Seaweeds and ulcerative colitis in laboratory animals. Lancet 2:489-490.
Mottet NK (1972) Editorial: On animal models for inflammatory bowel disease. Gastroenterology 62:1269-1271.

Onderdonk AB (1984). Role of intestinal microflora in Health and Disease 491-493.

Onderdonk AB and Bartlett JG (1979). Bacteriologic studies of experimental ulcerative colitis. Am J Clin Nutr 32:258-289.

Onderdonk AB, Cisneros RL and Bronson RT (1983). Enhancement of experimental ulcerative colitis by immunization with Bacteroides vulgatus. 783-788.

Onderdonk AB, Franklin ML, and Cisneros RL (1981). Production of experimental ulcerative colitis in gnotobiotic guinea pigs with simplified microflora. Infect Immun 32:225-231.

Onderdonk AB, Hermos JA, and Bartlett JG (1977). Role of intestinal microflora in experimental colitis. Am J Clin Nutr 32:1819-1825.

Onderdonk AB, Hermos JA, Dzink JL, and Bartlett JG (1978). Protective effect of metronidazole in experimental ulcerative colitis. Gastroenterology 74:521-526.

Oohashi Y, Ishioka T, Wakabayashi, and Kuwabara N (1981). A study on carcinogenesis induced by degraded carrageenan arising from squamous metaplasia of the rat colorectum. 267-272.

Oohashi Y, Kitamura S, Wakabayashi K, Kuwabara N, and Fukuda Y (1979). Irreversibility of degraded carrageenan-induced colorectal squamous metaplasia in rats. Gann, 70:391-392.

Shorter RG, Cardoza MR, Remine SG, Spencer RG, and Huizenga KA (1970a). Modification of in vitro cytotoxicity of lymphocytes from patients with chronic ulcerative colitis or granulomatous colitis for allogenic colonic epithelial cells. Gastroenterology 58:692-698.

Shorter RG, Huizenga KA, Remine SG, and Spencer RJ (1970b). Effects of preliminary incubation of lymphocytes with serum on their cytotoxicity for colonic epithelial cells. Gastroenterology 58:843-850.

Shorter RG, Huizenga KA, Spencer RJ, Aas J, and Guy SK (1971). Cytophilic antibody and the cytotoxicity of lymphocytes for colonic cells in vitro. Am J Dig Dis 16:673-680.

van der Waaij D, Cohen B, Anver M (1974). Mitagation of experimental inflammatory bowel disease in guinea pigs by selective elimination of the aerobic gram-negative intestinal microflora. Gastroenterology 67:460-472.

Wakabayashi K. Inagaki T, Jujimoto Y, and Fukuda Y (1978). Induction by degraded carrageenan of colorectal tumors in rats. Cancer Letters 4:171-176.

Watson DW (1969). Immune responses and the gut. Gastroenterology 56:944-965.

Watt J, Marcus R (1969). Ulcerative colitis in guinea
pigs caused by seaweed extract. J Pharm Pharmacol
21:1877-1885.

Watt J, Marcus R (1973). Progress report, experimental
ulcerative disease of the colon in animals. Gut
14:506-510.

Carcinoma of the Large Bowel and Its Precursors, pages 247–261
© **1985 Alan R. Liss, Inc.**

THE MARMOSET AS A MODEL OF ULCERATIVE COLITIS AND COLON CANCER

Neal K. Clapp, Clarence C. Lushbaugh,
Gretchen L. Humason, Barbara L. Gangaware,
Marsha A. Henke, and Arthur H. McArthur
Oak Ridge Associated Universities
Oak Ridge, TN 37831

INTRODUCTION

Colorectal cancer is one of the leading causes of death in the westernized countries of Europe, North America, Australia, and New Zealand. The American Cancer Society estimates that more than 130,000 new cases of colorectal cancer will be diagnosed annually in the United States (American Cancer Society 1984); this number is second only to the number of new cases of lung cancer. In addition, a large segment of the United States population is affected with inflammatory bowel disease. Prevalence rates indicate that 3% of all ulcerative colitis patients will ultimately develop colonic cancer. Risk for developing colonic cancer increases directly with duration of ulcerative colitis (1-2%/year) and with extent of colonic involvement (Lushbaugh et al 1977).

Most experimental studies of colon cancer use chemically-induced rodent models in which 1,2-dimethylhydrazine (DMH) or its metabolic derivatives produce a high incidence of colonic polyps and neoplasia. While this model system produces numerous polypoid lesions, differences exist between the relatively benign rodent tumors and the aggressive malignancies observed in humans. High incidences of spontaneous colonic carcinomas in the cotton-top tamarin, Saguinus oedipus oedipus, a small South American monkey (Clapp et al 1985a; Clapp et al 1985b; Lushbaugh et al 1977; Richter et al 1980), provide another animal model that can be studied to understand this disease process. Presumably, causative factors can be determined and manipulations of environmental factors and therapeutic agents can be studied which eventually may be applied to the human problem. Of particular interest is the fact that a colitis, which can become ulcerating during exacerbations, precedes and often accompanies the development of colon cancer in the cotton-top tamarin (Chalifoux, Bronson 1981; Lushbaugh et al 1985b). Further, two coexisting sister species, Saguinus fuscicollis illigeri (the saddle-back or white-lipped tamarin) and Callithrix jacchus (the common marmoset), develop a similar colitis but have not developed colon cancer in some 1500 necropsies over a 20-year period (Clapp et al 1985a; Clapp et al 1985b; Lushbaugh et al 1985a; Lushbaugh et al 1977; Richter et al 1980). Thus, we have an animal model for colon cancer which not only is spontaneous (not artificially induced), but also develops in the presence of colitis in the cancer-prone animal.

TAMARIN COLON CANCER

Tamarin colon cancer was first observed in 1967 and reported in 1978 at Oak Ridge Associated Universities (ORAU) (Lushbaugh et al 1977) and was subsequently confirmed in a second colony at New England Regional Primate Research Center (NERPRC) (Chalifoux, Bronson 1981). At this time, colon cancer has been reported in cotton-tops from four different colonies (Table 1).

TABLE 1
COLONIC CARCINOMAS DIAGNOSED IN
DIFFERENT *S.o. oedipus* COLONIES

Colony Site	Number of Cases
ORAU — (Oak Ridge)	81
— NCI (Formerly at Chicago)	3
NERPRC	29
BRISTOL, ENGL. (Epstein, Kirkwood)	1

In 1982, a tamarin colony from Rush Presbyterian-St. Luke's Medical Center, Chicago, was transferred to ORAU; prior to that time, colon cancer had not been reported in that colony. Three colonic carcinomas have been observed in those animals since the transfer; one case was diagnosed four months after the move. In addition, one colon tumor has been diagnosed in the S. o. oedipus colony at the University of Bristol, England (Dr. James Kirkwood, personal communication). Recently, we were also advised of a colon cancer diagnosed in a cotton-top from the Buffalo, NY, Zoological Gardens (Dr. Allen Prowten, personal communication). This wide geographic dispersion plus different environmental and husbandry protocols in use in these colonies suggest that this species has a genetic component to its cancer susceptibility.

At ORAU, colon carcinoma has been diagnosed in cotton-tops of both sexes and in both feral and colony-born animals. The mean time of occurrence was approximately 62 months of colony age (Clapp et al 1985a); however, this figure is increasing because some older animals have died with colon cancer. Tumors are located throughout the large bowel from cecum to rectum, but approximately 60% are found in the right side (cecum, ascending, and transverse colon). (Table 2).

TABLE 2
LOCATION OF 81 PRIMARY CARCINOMAS
OF THE LARGE BOWEL *(S.o. oedipus)*

NUMBER OF ANIMALS	81
CECUM	41
ASCENDING COLON	37
TRANSVERSE COLON	29
DESCENDING COLON	46
RECTUM	13
NOS	3
MULTIPLES	49

Most of the cancers are multicentric and some animals have numerous primary foci of comparable size throughout the large bowel (Clapp et al 1985a; Clapp et al 1985b; Lushbaugh et al 1985b; Lushbaugh et al 1977; Richter et al 1980). The similarity between these observations of multiple primary cancers in cotton-top tamarins with colitis and those in human patients with longstanding ulcerative colitis and multiple malignant primaries throughout the colon is intriguing (Goulston, McGovern 1981; Dr. Owen Peck, U. of Nevada School of Medicine, personal communication).

Prior to 1981, colon cancer in tamarins had not been observed in ORAU animals which were >7 years of colony age (Clapp et al 1985a) Since 1981, a number of older tamarins (9-13 years of age) died with colonic cancer; some of them were colony-born of known ages. Since 1976, ORAU has not imported any cotton-top tamarins because of their endangered species status; consequently, the colony composition has changed from predominantly feral to pre-dominantly colony-born. In spite of this population shift, most of the colon cancer deaths have occurred between 3-8 years of colony age. Table 3 shows the fraction of deaths due to colon cancer by age from 1981 to 1984.

TABLE 3
FREQUENCY OF COLONIC CARCINOMAS IN
RECENT *S.o. oedipus* DEATHS

Year of Deaths	Colony Age (No. Cancers/No. Deaths)		
	(1-3 years)	*(4-7 years)*	*(≥ 8 years)*
1981	0/1	15/19	2/3
1982	0/0	8/13	2/5
1983	1/8	6/9	2/5
1984	0/1	4/6	0/2

(7/15/84)

Since 1981, 60% of animals dying ≥ 4 years of colony age have had colon cancer. Because colon cancer has been observed in only one of three co-habiting species, a strong genetic component is suggested.

TAMARIN COLITIS

Each of the three co-habiting species develop colitis which may ulcerate and which is observed prior to and during the development of colon cancer in S. o. oedipus. Clinically, chronic diarrhea with accompanying weight loss has been observed in numerous tamarins over periods of several months, with and without occult blood; morbidity and severity of diarrhea in the ORAU colony have been reduced in recent years with improved nutritional and husbandry practices. Parasitism, which was common in imported animals, and enteric microbial infections are relatively uncommon as causes of diarrhea. Likewise, wasting marmoset disease, which has been reported in most marmoset colonies, is now essentially nonexistent in the ORAU colony. Currently, when an S. o. oedipus suffers weight loss and chronic diarrhea, the most common etiology has been colon cancer.

MATERIALS AND METHODS

Two approaches were considered in the evaluation of colitis in the ORAU colony. Necropsy tissues from several hundred colons of several species are readily available; and biopsy tissues can be obtained from living animals. Recent deaths (from 1979-84) were selected for retrospective examination since most of these animals have been necropsied promptly after death, several have been euthanized when moribund, and, generally, the tissues from these animals have minimal autolysis. Animals were grouped by possible factors that might contribute to marmoset colitis as shown in Table 4.

All groups were age-matched in the three species (≥ 10 animals/group), excepting colon cancer animals which occurred in S. o. oedipus only. After the animals were selected, the identifying animal numbers on the histology slides were covered and coded. All groups were randomized and examined blindly and data were recorded. After

TABLE 4
TAMARIN AND MARMOSET GROUPS EXAMINED FOR COLITIS

Effects Considered	Animal Groups Studied
1. AGE AT DEATH (Young vs. Adult)	COLONY-BORN THAT DIED <1 YEAR OF AGE VS. COLONY-BORN THAT DIED >1 YEAR
2. SOURCE OF ANIMALS	COLONY-BORN VS. IMPORTS
3. DEATH	ANIMALS THAT DIED VS. THOSE THAT WERE EUTHANIZED
4. COLON CANCER	*S.o. oedipus* WITH COLON CANCER VS. NONCOLON CANCER

the histological evaluation of all groups was completed, the data were decoded and information compiled by groups. A total of 118 animals were examined retrospectively and included 64 S. o. oedipus, 30 S. f. illigeri, and 24 C. jacchus.

The numbers and types of cells infiltrating into the epithelium and lamina propria were counted and epithelial and crypt changes were noted (Table 5).

TABLE 5
CRITERIA FOR EVALUATING CELLULAR INFILTRATE

		Numbers of Cells			
		PMN's			
Score	Epith. (per crypt)	Lam. Prop.	Plasma Cells	Mononuclear	Lymphocytes
0	0	0–1	<5	<5	<5
1	1	2–5	10–25	10–25	10–25
2	2–3	10–20	50–75	50–75	50–75
3	>5	Focal Clusters	>100	>100	>100

Each colonic segment (cecum, ascending, transverse, and descending) was evaluated. First, the entire segment (which had been fixed and imbedded in paraffin in a "Swiss roll") was examined and any unusual observations were recorded. To determine a consistent location for scoring, the mid-point of the segment was then approximated. The area selected for evaluation was required to be representative of the entire segment. Then, 2-3 crypts and associated lamina propria were evaluated; cells were identified (400X) and counted (250X). The assigned activity grade for each colonic segment was expressed by:

1) a letter

N = Normal
A = Acute
S = Subacute
C = Chronic

and 2) a number

1 = Mild
2 = Moderate
3 = Severe

The colon activity grade was determined as follows: When chronic inflammatory cells (plasma cells, lymphocytes, and histiocytes) were predominant, the activity was designated chronic (or C). If, in addition to chronic inflammatory cells, some polymorphonuclear leukocytes (PMN's) were present in the lamina propria and/or the epithelium, or an occasional crypt abscess was present, subacute (or S) was assigned. When the infiltrate included an abundance of PMN's (including microabcesses) in the lamina propria and/or crypt epithelium and crypt abscesses were common, the condition was considered as acute (or A). The accompanying numbers (1, 2, or 3) were given to describe the severity (i.e., mild, moderate, or severe, respectively). Any differences in inflammatory activity from that seen at the mid-point of the segment were also recorded.

RESULTS AND DISCUSSION

Most of the animals (deaths from 1979-84) had a mild chronic colitis regardless of species or variable (Table 4) considered. Only a few colons were considered "normal" with "test-tube"-like crypts which were in close apposition to each other and with essentially no cellular infiltrate in the lamina propria (Figure 1).

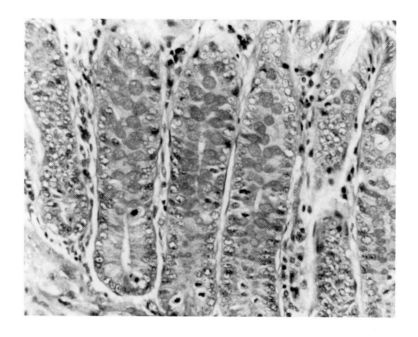

FIGURE 1:   "Normal" crypts of Leiberkuhn in a marmoset
colon.   Note   "test-tube"-like   crypts   with
essentially   no   cellular   infiltrate   in   the
lamina propria. PAS. 100 X.

In   most   colons,   the   inflammatory   activity   was
relatively consistent from the cecum through the rectum,
and a single score was adequate to describe the inflammatory   state.   These   observations   contrast   with   the
occurrence of ulcerative colitis in humans in which the
lesion is usually most severe in the rectum and less
severe with increasing distance retrograde from the anus
(Goulston, McGovern 1981).   In chronic tamarin colitis
(Figure 2), crypts were often atrophic (in length and
number)   with   an   increased   itercrypt   space,   crypt
distortions and malformations were common.

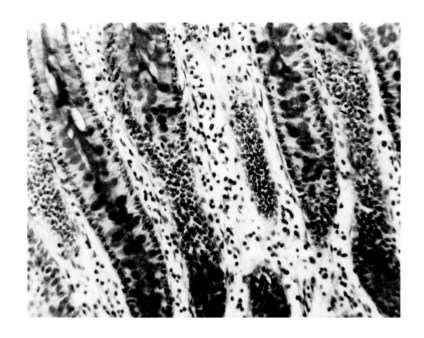

FIGURE   2: Chronic   colitis   in   a   tamarin.   Cellular
           infiltrate into the lamina propria consisted
           primarily   of   plasma   cells,   lymphocytes,
           histiocytes, and other mononuclear cells.   PAS
           100X.

    Since these were retrospective studies, progressive
stages   of   the   disease   process   were   not   identified.
However, acute colitis was characterized by large numbers
of PMN's in the lamina propria; often these accumulated to
form microabscesses (Figure 3).

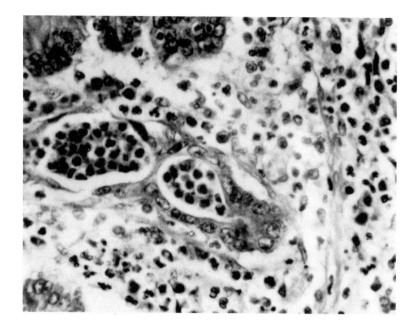

FIGURE 3: Acute tamarin colitis. Polymorphonuclear cells
(PMN's) were concentrated in the lamina
propria. Crypts show mucin depletion. PAS,
250X.

PMN's infiltrated into the crypt epithelium (Figure 4)
often in large numbers, and eventually reached the crypt
lumen to form crypt abscesses.

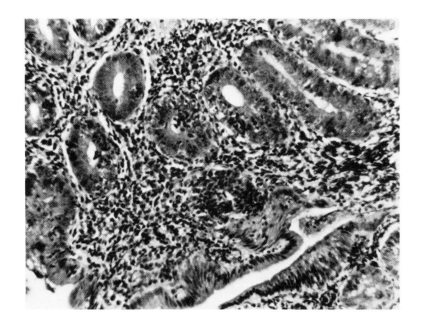

FIGURE 4: Acute tamarin colitis in a rectal biopsy. Large numbers of PMN's were seen in several crypts. PAS, 250X.

Crypt abscesses were seen adjacent to crypts with mild chronic cellular infiltrate extending into the lamina propria (Figure 5); this finding may suggest that crypt abscesses were an end-stage of the acute inflammatory process as remission occurred.

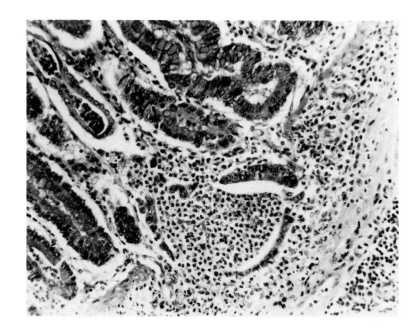

FIGURE 5: Crypt abscess that appeared to have "ruptured",
releasing PMN's into lamina propria. Adjacent
lamina propria was scored as mild chronic
colitis. PAS 100X.

Ulceration was frequent and often multiple; however,
evidence of severe hemorrhagic episodes as described in
human ulcerative colitis (Goulston, McGovern 1981) was not
seen. An extensive desmoplastic response on the serosal
surface frequently accompanied mucosal ulceration.

The contribution of each variable to tamarin colitis
has not yet been determined. However, some preliminary
observations have been made. In most of the examined
groups, one or more animals had acute colitis that was
either moderate or severe and was in one or more colonic

segments. The cause of these inflammatory exacerbations was not obvious. More severe cases of acute colitis were found in the S. o. oedipus group which had colon cancer; however, even in this group, there were some animals with cancer and a mild chronic inflammation throughout the colon. Animals with cancer and mild chronic colitis often had smaller primary tumors. This suggests that severe acute colitis may occur either as a complication of colon cancer growth or as a possible promoter of initiated cells to cause cancer expression. It was not uncommon to observe in situ primary tumors immediately adjacent to crypts graded as mild chronic colitis.

Dysplasia, as associated with human inflammatory bowel disease (Riddell et al 1984), was not recognized by the authors or by Dr. John Yardley (1985) or other pathologists who examined ORAU tamarin tissues prior to a workshop to discuss the marmoset as a model for human colon disease (ORAU-NIH sponsored workshop 1984). In tamarin colitis, hyperplasia of the crypt epithelium was common with stratification of nuclei, but nuclear hyperchromatism was uncommon. The observation that "neoplastic transformation in the marmoset was markedly dedifferentiated from the outset" (Yardley 1985) suggest that some differences exist in colon cancer onset between tamarins and humans; carcinoma in situ may be the rule in tamarin colon cancer rather than the exception as reported in humans. However, nuclear hyperplasia, mucin depletion, dystrophic mucin cells, and abnormal crypt morphology were common epithelial changes in the tamarin inflammatory process and accompanied colon cancer development in S. o. oedipus.

Preliminary information has been obtained about variables that might modify the prevalence or severity of colitis and ultimately of colon cancer, but the cause-effect relationship remains unanswered. This retrospective study of necropsy tissues evaluated only animals which died; causes of death may or may not have been related to the state of the colon. Systematic biopsies of cotton-tops as they enter into and continue through the very high-risk ages of 3-8 years and of age-matched non-susceptible tamarins and marmosets should provide information about the cause and effect relationship of the two diseases. Ultimately, preventive and therapeutic measures may be evaluated for both colitis and colon cancer in tamarins. Similarities between tamarin and human colon disease may then be compared, and protocols which are effective in the animal model may be employed in diagnosis, management, and preventive measures in humans.

ACKNOWLEDGEMENT

This work is based on work currently supported by Oak Ridge Associated Universities Corporation and National Cancer Institute, DHHS, Contract No. NO1 CP 21004.

REFERENCES

Chalifoux LV, Bronson RT (1981). Colonic adenocarcinoma associated with chronic colitis in cotton-top marmosets, Satuinus oedipus. Gastroenterology 80:942-946.

Clapp NK, Lushbaugh CC, Humason GL, Gangaware BL, Henke MA (1985a). Natural history and pathology of colon cancer in Saguinus oedipus oedipus. Dig. Dis. Sci. (in press)

Clapp NK, LushbaughCC, Humason GL, Gangaware BL, Henke MA (1985b). The cotton-top tamarin as an animal model of colorectal cancer metastasis. In: The Biology and Treatment of Colorectal Cancer Metastasis Martinus Nijhoff Publishing, Hingham, MA. (in press).

Goulston SJM, McGovern VS (1981). Fundamentals of colitis. Pergamon Press, Sydney, Australia.

Lushbaugh CC, Humason GL, Clapp NK (1985a). Histology of colitis: Saguinus oedipus oedipus and other marmosets. Dig. Dis. Sci. (in press).

Lushbaugh CC, Humason GL, Clapp NK (1985b). Histology of colon cancer in Saguinus oedipus oedipus. Dig. Dis. Sci. (in press).

Lushbaugh CC, Humason GL, Swartzendruber DC, Richter CB, Gengozian N (1977). Spontaneous colonic adenocarcinoma in marmosets. Proceedings of the Conference, Oak Ridge, TN 1977. In: Gengozian N, Dienhardt F (eds) Primates Med (10): Basel, Karger, 1978, pp 119-134.

ORAU-NIH Sponsored workshop (1984). "Is the marmoset an experimental model to study gastrointestinal disease?" Oak Ridge Associated Universities, Oak Ridge, TN, Dig Dis Sci, April 18-20, 1984.

Richter CB, Lushbaugh CC, Swartzendruber DC (1980). Cancer of the colon in cotton-top tamarins. In: Montali RJ, Migaki G (eds) Comp Pathol Zoo Anim: pp 567-571.

Riddell RH, Goldman H, Rausohoff DF, Appelman HD, Fenoglio CM, Haggitt RC, Ahren C, Correa P, Hamilton SR, Morson BC, Sommers SC, and Yardley JH (1984). Dysplasia in inflammatory bowel disease: Standardized classification with provisional clinical applications. Human Path 14:931-968.
Yardley JH (1985). Comments on the comparative pathology of colonic neoplasia in the cotton-top marmoset (Saguinus oedipus oedipus). Dig. Dis. Sci. (in press).

Carcinoma of the Large Bowel and Its Precursors, pages 263-276
© 1985 Alan R. Liss, Inc.

BIOCHEMICAL APPROACHES TO THE INTERVENTION OF LARGE BOWEL CANCER

Michael J. Hill, Ph.D.
Director, Bacterial Metabolism Research Lab.
Public Health Laboratory Service Center for
    Applied Microbiology and Research
Salisbury, U.K.

INTRODUCTION

In 1975 we published the results of a case-control study of colorectal cancer which suggested that the combination of high fecal bile acid (high FBA) concentration and carriage of the clostridia able to desaturate the steroid nucleus (NDC) was associated with the disease (Hill et al 1975). In that study the control persons were patients with non- malignant bowel disease since it was believed that bowel disease causes a modification of the diet (in terms of total food intake as well as type of food) and, since the FBA concentration is related to diet, it was essential to control for the presence of bowel disease per se. There have been a number of studies purporting to attempt to repeat our study but all used healthy control persons and so failed to control for the change in diet associated with gut disease. The report by Moskwitz et al (1978) prompted us to segregate our patient series (now extended to more than 100) into various Dukes classes; we also segregated the patients by tumor subsite (Hill 1981) and compared them with healthy control persons. "High FBA" concentration was classified as being above the 80 percentile point of the distribution in the controls (as in our original study, Hill et al 1975) so that 8% of our control persons had the combination of high FBA and carriage of NDC. When analyzed in this way (Table 1), there was still a clear discrimination between the healthy controls and persons with Dukes A or B cancers of the left colon or rectum, but only a poor discrimination for cancers of the right and

Table 1
Fecal analyses in persons with colorectal cancer and in healthy control persons.

	Number assayed	Mean FBA concentration (mg/g. dry wt)	% carrying NDC	% with high ± FBA/NDC+
Healthy control persons	100	7.9	38%	10%
All colorectal cancer cases	120	10.4	79%	50%
Dukes' A cases	17	10.6	88%	77%
Dukes' B cases	36	10.7	72%	52%
Dukes' C cases	28	9.5	80%	32%
Patients with liver metastases	10	6.8	30%	0%
All colon cancers*	37	10.6	80%	47%
Cecum + Asc. + Trans.*	17	8.3	80%	22%
Desc. + sigmoid*	20	11.4	80%	55%
All rectal cancers*	38	10.3	79%	58%

* Contain no cases which have liver metastases.
± "high FBA" includes those above the 80th percentile of the normal population (which currently is 9.9 mg/g dry weight).
FBA = fecal bile acid.
NDC = nuclear dehydrating clostridia.

transverse colon and an inverse correlation for colon cancers with liver metastases. Our larger group of patients was selected to try to exclude Dukes' C cases, since we wished to follow-up this group of high-risk patients as described later. Most of the patients were from St. Mark's Hospital which, for various reasons, has an abnormally high proportion of cancers of the left colon and rectum. Thus, by fortuitous patient selection (with a very low proportion of Dukes' C and of right colon cancers) and deliberate selection of controls (with non-malignant disease), we achieved a result indicating discrimination between the fecal analyses of bowel cancer cases and controls that was not found by others. After the further analysis of the results described above, we remain convinced that the results suggest a role for bile acid metabolites in bowel carcinogenesis; however, we accept that the fecal analyses described are unlikely to be of assistance in selecting persons from the general population at high risk of the disease.

Since that study we have attempted to amplify our understanding of bowel carcinogenesis by the study of high risk patient groups. These studies have been conducted in parallel with a large prospective study of 8,000 persons, the results of which are due to be analyzed in late 1985. In this presentation I will discuss the results of studies of the high risk patient groups.

FOLLOW-UP OF LARGE BOWEL CANCER CASES

Patients who have been successfully treated for large bowel cancer are at increased risk of developing another primary carcinoma in the colorectal remnant. The overall excess risk is thought to be 3 to 6 fold and is greater if there were adenomas in addition to the carcinoma in the resected specimen (Polk et al 1965). We have therefore assembled a cohort of 110 patients who have been treated by resection of tumor and anastomosis to give a normal excretory action. Of these patients 39 had at least one adenoma in addition to the carcinoma at the time of diagnosis (C+A) while the remaining 71 had a solitary carcinoma (C-A). It was hoped that this group of patients could be studied prospectively to determine the relation between fecal analyses and the risk of subsequent colorectal cancer development.

The patients have been followed since 1974, but because they have been followed clinically, and all adenomas removed when detected, there have been no cancers in this group of patients (which would be expected if the adenoma-carcinoma sequence is the major route of colo-rectal carcinogenesis). We have therefore been unable to analyze the results in the way that was originally intended.

Of the cohort of patients, 50% had "high risk" fecal analyses (high FBA and carriage of NDC), 50% for C+A, and 50% for C-A; immediately postoperatively there was a sharp decrease in FBA concentration and loss of NDC in 63% of the patients followed by a recovery period, so that 12 months postoperation the fecal analyses had returned to a new "steady state". The "steady" postoperative fecal analyses were then assessed to see whether they suggested a "high risk" of colorectal cancer or a "low risk"; 35% of the total group were assessed as "high risk" suggesting a 4-fold excess risk in comparison with the normal popula-tion, and when divided into the two groups, the C+A group contained 52% "high risk" (6-fold excess risk) while the C-A group contained 25% "high risk" (suggesting only 3-fold excess risk of the disease).

PATIENTS WITH COLORECTAL ADENOMAS

The adenoma-carcinoma sequence in colorectal carcino-genesis has, in recent years, been modified to the dysplasia-carcinoma sequence (Morson, Konishi 1981) to make it compatible with the dysplasia-carcinoma observed at other sites (eg, the uterine cervix, the stomach, etc.). Although under most circumstances dysplasia of the colonic mucosa is manifest as a raised polyp or an adenoma, this revision now takes account of the situation where dysplasia is usually not manifest as an adenoma. This is common in ulcerative colitis and presumably occurs on occasion in the normal colon, although it is rarely detected.

Since adenomas are removed when detected, there has been an opportunity to carry out studies of the relation between fecal analyses and the rate of growth of an adenoma or the rate of increase in the severity of epithelial dysplasia. However, we have attempted to determine the role of FBA AND NDC in the various stages of colorectal carcinogenesis illustrated in Figure 1. We have analyzed fecal samples from 133 patients with colorectal adenomas, 22 patients with non-adenomatous polyps (eg, hyperplastic polyps, fibrous polyps, juvenile polyps, etc.) and compared them with an age- and sex-matched group of healthy persons living in South Wales who were part of another study.

Figure 1
Postulated mechanism for the adenoma-carcinoma sequence

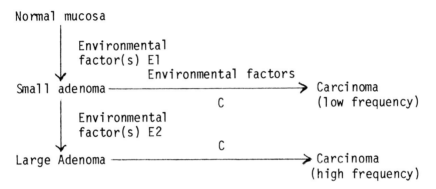

When the patients with adenomatous polyps were compared with the healthy controls there was no difference in the fecal analyses (Table 2); further, there was no relation between the number of adenomas detected in these patients during the period 1974-1984 and the fecal analyses. Thus, it is clear that there is no role for FBA or NDC in the initial formation of a small adenoma (Factor E1). When the group of patients with adenomas was subdivided on the basis of the severity of epithelial dysplasia of the most severely dysplastic adenoma there was a correlation between this and the FBA concentration and carriage rate of NDC. This suggests that a bacterial metabolite of bile acids might be important in determining both the rate of growth of an adenoma (Factor E2) and the rate of increase in severity of epithelial dysplasia (Factor C).

It is of interest to note that in our studies the fecal analyses of patients with large adenomas (especially large villous adenomas) or with severely dysplastic

Table 2

Fecal analyses in patients with colorectal adenomas

	Number of patients	Mean FBA concentration (mg/g dry wt)	% carrying NDC
Control persons	100	8.7±2.5	38%
Non-adenomatous polyps	22	6.9±1.2	38%
Adenoma patients	133	8.8±2.2	42%
Adenomas > 20mm diam.	32	11.4±2.4	70%
10-20mm	45	8.0±2.6	45%
5-10mm	30	7.9±1.5	37%
< 5mm	26	6.7±1.2	7%
Adenomas with mild dysplasia	84	8.3±2.4	38%
Moderate or severe dysplasia	39	10.0±2.1	49%

adenomas are very similar to those of patients with Dukes' A colorectal cancer. These are the major factors in conferring malignant potential on an adenoma; just as there is a spectrum of histological features in an adenoma (either in size or in dysplasia), so there is also a spectrum of fecal analyses which is correlated with the histopathology.

In studying high-risk patient groups it is important to remember that, since more than 50% of men aged 70 years or more at autopsy are found to carry colorectal adenomas (Williams et al 1982), carriage of adenomas does not, per se, confer a high risk; a high risk is associated with carriage of large adenomas. Thus, it was not surprising that there was no difference in fecal analyses between all adenoma patients and controls in this study and in two other reports (Mudd et al 1978; Tanida et al 1984); this would be expected whether or not bile acids were important in colorectal carcinogenesis. In attempting to determine the role of fecal components in colorectal carcinogenesis by studying adenoma patients, it is essential to have full clinical/histopathological information (size, villous component, dysplasia, sub-site, etc.) on all of the adenomas.

CHRONIC ULCERATIVE COLITIS

Ulcerative colitis of the large bowel carries a high risk of colorectal cancer if it is of longstanding duration. The factors determining the magnitude of the risk were studied in detail by MacDougall (1964) who showed that the risk was maximum if the age of onset was less than 30, the disease involved the whole of the large bowel, and if the duration of the disease was more than 10 years. The policy at St. Mark's Hospital with patients having pan-colitis of more than 10-years duration is to offer and advise a total colectomy and, to those who refuse this advice, to offer regular clinical examination of the large bowel for pre-cancerous changes in the epithelial mucosa. In those patients in whom pre-cancer is detected in biopsies from the rectum or sigmoid colon, a prophylactic total colectomy is strongly urged and the resected specimen often already contains carcinoma. However, in almost all cases, carcinoma has been limnited to the mucosa and to date there have been no deaths from

Table 3

Fecal analyses in patients with ulcerative colitis of more than 10-years duration involving the whole colon, and in control persons.

	Number of patients	Mean FBA concentration (mg/g dry wt)	Proportion of persons carrying NDC
Healthy control persons	100	8.7	38%
Persons with ulcerative colitis	112	8.2	30%
Those with no dysplasia	68	7.9	30%
Those with dysplasia	44	8.7	30%
mild	22	7.4	29%
moderate	8	9.5	13%
severe	14	10.5	43%
Lost to the study - dead	6	5.7	0%
- colectomy	9	6.9	25%

cancer in this group of patients (Lennard-Jones et al 1977).

We have studied the fecal steroids and bacteria in 112 such patients (Table 3). We began recruiting into this group in 1974 and all 112 patients have been studied for 5 to 10 years. During that time, 6 have died and so have been lost to the study, and a further 9 have suffered a severe relapse in their symptoms of colitis and for this reason had a total colectomy and so were also lost to the study. Of the remainder, 44 developed epithelial dysplasia which has remained mild in 22, moderately severe in 8, and severe in 14; severe dysplasia is the signal for surgery and of those patients, 10 had a carcinoma (all Dukes' A).

When the 112 patients were considered as a group, both mean FBA concentration and the carriage rate of NDC were low when compared with the normal population. In these patients dysplasia remains in the plane of the mucosa and only rarely is manifest as a raised lump. However, the dysplasia cases can be accepted as being equivalent to adenomas, so that analysis of this patient group was similar to that in the adenoma patients. Thus, the group of 44 patients with dysplasia had fecal analyses very similar to the total group of patients, indicating that bile acids and NDC play no role in this stage of carcinogenesis. When the patients were grouped on the basis of the severity of their epithelial dysplasia, there is a clear relation between this and the fecal analyses (Table 3).

These results support the suggestion that although bile acid metabolites play no role in the initiation of dysplasia they promote its progession to carcinoma. The results differ from those of Reddy et al (1974), who found an increased FBA concentration in colitis. It is impossible to compare the two sets of data because Reddy et al gave no clinical information on the severity, duration, and extent of the disease in their patients.

IMPROVEMENT OF THE FBA/NDC DISCRIMINANT

We have attempted to improve the discriminant value of the combination of high FBA/carriage of NDC by (a) testing the value of individual bile acids in comparison with the concentration of total FBA, (b) the assay of the hydrogen acceptor which permit the NDC to desaturate the steroid nucleus, and (c) testing for further bile acid degrading enzymes.

We have assayed cholanoyl 7-dehydroxylase activity in the feces of large bowel cancer cases and control persons and have confirmed the results of Mastromarino et al (1976). However, it was necessary to carry out the assay on fresh stool samples collected in bacteria-protective medium; until the assay has been modified to make it more robust, it is not suitable for epidemiological studies of large numbers of samples.

We have identified the hydrogen acceptor necessary for the desaturation of the bile acid nucleus by NDC as a quinone (Fernandez and Hill, 1975, 1978) probably menaquinone (vitamin K). The menaquinones in feces are of bacterial and of dietary origin; the latter (phylloquinone) is relatively easy to assay but there are technical difficulties associated with the quantitative assay of bacterial menaquinones because of their great variety; however, the studies by Fernandez et al (1984) suggest that the major menaquinones in feces should be MK9 to MK12 (those produced by the Bacteroides fragilis group of organisms) since the other organisms either do not produce menaquinones or are so greatly outnumbered by the Bacteroides species that their menaquinones are quantitatively insignificant. Methods for the assay of fecal menaquinones have been developed and the discriminant value of fecal menaquinone assays either alone or in combination with the FBA/NDC discriminant is being assessed.

Our initial studies of the individual bile acids have been concentrated on lithocholic acid (LA) and deoxycholic acid (DCA) since these are the two that have been shown to have tumor promoting activity. Our results to date suggest that the ratio of LA:DCA is a much better discriminant that total FBA, LA, or DCA alone; the evidence in support of this has been summarized by Owen et al (1983; 1984) and Thompson et al (1984). The results made no sense until Wilpart et al (1983, 1984) reported that in co-mutagenesis assays LA and DCA were antagonistic when present in comparable amounts and that a large excess of either acid was necessary for co-mutagenis activity. In practice we rarely find the necessary large excess of DCA and large excesses of LA are much more common. We are currently examining the discriminant value of LA/DCA in combination with NDC carriage.

CONCLUSIONS

The evidence incriminating bile acids in colorectal carcinogenesis is growing; in summary:

(a) Some of the major fecal bile acids have been shown to be cocarcinogenic in the rodent colon and comutagenic in the Salmonella mutagenesis assay system (Narisawa et al 1974; Wilpart et al 1983);

(b) Bile acid receptors have been detected in the mucosa of 31% of bowel cancer cases, but only 2.4% of control persons (Summerton et al 1984);

(c) Bile acid turnover is faster in patients with colo-rectal adenomas than in control persons and colonic absorption of bile acids is faster in adenoma cases than in controls (Van der Werf et al 1983);

(d) The FBA concentration is correlated with the inci-dence of cancer in populations (Hill et al 1971; Reddy et al 1973; Hill et al 1982) and with the malignant potential of adenomas of various size and severity of dysplasia;

(e) In a case-control study, the FBA concentration discri- minates between controls and cases of early cancer of the left colon and rectum, but not cases of cancer of the right colon or cases of advanced metastatic disease;

(f) In patients with ulcerative colitis involving the whole colon for more than 10 years, the FBA concentration was higher in those who went on to develop severe dyspla-sia or carcinoma than in those who remained free of dysplasia.

However, although the evidence suggests that bile acids are important in colorectal cancer during the promotion phase, increasing the risk of a small adenoma (with low malignant potential) growing to a large size (with much greater risk of malignancy) and increasing the severity of epithelial dysplasia in adenomatous tissues, our understanding of their role has not yet reached the stage where they can be used to predict who is at high risk of the disease. Our current knowledge is more likely to be of value in the near future in helping to prevent colon carcinogenesis in patients with ulcerative colitis of long duration.

ACKNOWLEDGEMENT

This work is financially supported by the Cancer Research Campaign.

REFERENCES

Fernandez F, Hill MJ (1975). The production of vitamin K by human intestinal bacteria. J. Med Microbiol 8: Pix.

Fernandez F, Hill MJ (1978). A faecal hydrogen acceptor for clostridial 3-oxo steroid $^{\Delta}4$-dehydrogenase. Biochem Soc Trans 6:376.

Fernandez F, Collins MD, Hill MJ (1984). Production of vitamin K by human gut bacteria. Biochem Soc Trans (in press).

Hill MJ, Drasar BS, Aries VC, Crowther JS, Hawksworth GM, Willaims REO (1971). Bacteria and etiology of cancer of the large bowel. Lancet 1:95.

Hill MJ, Drasar BS, Williams REO, Meade TW, Cox AG, Simpson JEP, Morson BC (1975). Faecal bile acids and clostridia in patients with cancer of the large bowel. Lancet 1:535.

Hill MJ, Taylor AJ, Thompson MH, Wait R (1982). Faecal steroids and urinary volatile phenols in four Scandinavian populations. Nutr Cancer 4:67.

Lennard-Jones J, Morson BC, Ritchie JK, Shove D, Williams CB (1977). Cancer in colitis: assessment of the individual risk by clinical and histological criteria. Gastroenterology 73:1280.

MacDougall IPM (1964). The cancer risk in ulcerative colitis. Lancet 2:655.

Mastromarino A, Reddy BS, Wynder EL (1976). Metabolic epidemiology of colon cancer: enzymic activities of the faecal flora. Am J Clin Nutr 29:1455.

Morson BS, Konishi F (1980). Dysplasia of the colorectum. In Wright R (ed) "Recent Advances in Gastrointestinal Pathology" London W B Saunders, p331.

Moskwitz M, White C, Floch M (1978). Bile acid and neutral steroid excretion in carcinoma of the colon, other cancers and control subjects. Gastroenterology 75:1071.

Mudd DG, McKelvey ST, Sloan JM, Elmore DT (1978). Faecal bile acid concentrations in patients at increased risk of large bowel cancer. Act Gastro Belg 41:241.

Narisawa T, Magadia N, Weisburger J, Wynder EL (1974). Promoting effect of bile acids on colon carcinogenesis after intrarectal instillation N-methyl-N-nitro-N-nitrosoquanidine in rats. J Nat Cancer Inst 53:1093.

Owen RW, Dodo M, Thompson MH, Hill MJ (1983). The faecal ratio of lithocholic acid to deoxycholic acid may be an important aetiological factor in colorectal cancer. Eur J Cancer Clin Oncol 19:1307.

Owen RW, Dodo M, Thompson MH, Hill MJ (1984). The faecal ratio of lithocholic acid to deoxycholic acid may be an important aetiological factor in colorectal cancer. Biochem Soc Trans 12:861.

Polk HC, Spratt JS, Butcher HR (1965). Frequence of multiple primary malignant neoplasm associated with colorectal carcinoma. Am J Surg 109:71.

Reddy BS, Wynder EL 1973). Large bowel carcinogenesis: faecal constituents of populations with diverse incidence of colon cancer. J Nat Cancer Inst 50:1437.

Reddy BS, Martin CW, Wynder EL (1974). Fecal file acids and cholesterol metabolites of patients with ulcerative colitis, a high risk group for development of colon cancer. Cancer Res 37:1697.

Summerton J, Flynn M, Cooke T, Taylor I (1984). Bile acid receptors in colorectal cancer. Br J Surg 70:549.

Tanida N, Hikasa Y, Shimoyama T, Setchell K (1984). Comparison of fecal bile acid profiles between patients with adenomatous polyps of the large bowel and healthy subjects in Japan. Gut 25:824.

Thompson MH, Owen RW, Cummings JC, Hill MJ (1984). Factors affecting faecal bile acid concentrations: fat and fibre. Biochem Soc Trans (in press).

Van Der Werf SD, Nagengast FM, Van Berge Henegouwan GP, Huijbregts AW, Van Tongeren JH (1983). Intracolonic environment and the presence of colonic adenomas in man. Gut 24:876.

Williams AR, Balasooriya BA, Day DW (1982). Polyps and cancer of the large bowel: a necropsy study in Liverpool. Gut 23:835.

Wilpart M, Mainguet P, Maskens A, Roberfroid M (1983)
Mutagenicity of 1,2-dimethylhydrazine towards Salmonella
typhimurium. Carcinogenesis 4:45.

Wilpart M, Mainguet P, Maskens A, Roberfroid M (1984)
Structure activity relationships among biliary acids
showing co-mutagenic activity towards 1,2-dimethylhy-
drazine. Carcinogenesis 5:1239.

Carcinoma of the Large Bowel and Its Precursors, pages 277–284
© 1985 Alan R. Liss, Inc.

DIETARY APPROACHES TO THE PREVENTION OF LARGE BOWEL CANCER

Gail E. McKeown-Eyssen, Ph.D., Epidemiologist
Ludwig Institute for Cancer Research
Toronto, Ontario, CANADA, and
Associate Professor, Department of Preventive
Medicine & Biostatistics, University of Toronto

That diet may play a role in the etiology of human colon cancer has been suggested by strong correlations between national incidence or mortality from colon cancer and national levels of availability of foods. Unfortunately, dietary hypotheses have not received strong or consistent support from case-control or cohort studies designed to test them. For example, national availability of dietary fat is highly correlated with colon cancer incidence and mortality (Armstrong and Doll 1975, Knox 1977), yet case-control studies focusing on consumption of high fat foods have provided mixed results. Increased relative risk of colon cancer has been found to be associated with high total fat consumption (Jain et al 1980), and with consumption of foods high in saturated fats (Phillips 1975), but three additional studies (Dales et al 1978, Modan et al 1975, Higginson 1966) found no significant association with consumption of high saturated fat foods and no association has been seen with consumption of fried foods (Graham et al 1978, Higginson 1966, Phillips 1975, Wynder et al 1969). The lack of consistent findings does not necessarily mediate against a dietary etiology of colon cancer, however, the findings may have arisen, at least in part, from methodological limitations of the studies (McKeown-Eyssen and Bruce, unpublished data). Accurate assessment of diet is difficult, especially when diet before the onset of disease must be recalled. In addition, diet within a community may be relatively homogeneous and where there is little range in consumption, and therefore little range in risk, it may be difficult to detect associations between diet and disease in studies of practical size (McKeown-Eyssen and Thomas, unpublished data).

RANDOMIZED TRIALS OF DIETARY INTERVENTIONS

One means of avoiding the methodologic limitations of observational epidemiologic studies is to test the dietary hypotheses by the strongest epidemiological study design, the randomized trial. In such trials, participants are allocated at random into one or more study groups, each of which receives a diet or a dietary supplement which is hypothesized to reduce the risk of cancer, or into a 'control' group which maintains a 'normal' diet or receives a placebo supplement. Compliance to the intervention is monitored and, after a suitable period, the groups are compared in terms of a clinical outcome.

CLINICAL OUTCOMES FOR RANDOMIZED TRIALS

The duration of a trial, and the number of participants required, will depend on the rate of occurrence of the chosen outcome. Cancer incidence or mortality is clearly the outcome of ultimate interest but trials of this nature require the study of many thousands of persons over a number of years (Bruce et al 1981). The feasibility of such a trial will depend heavily on the type of dietary intervention planned. Where a dietary supplement, such as vitamins, can be taken easily, participants can be provided with the necessary pills and reasonable compliance might be expected over a number of years with relatively little contact with the study team. Where the dietary intervention requires a major alteration in diet, such as reduction in the total fat consumed, frequent, perhaps monthly, dietary counseling may be necessary to achieve adequate compliance and this is impractical if thousands of participants must be followed for a number of years. Alternative endpoints have been sought which occur at a sufficiently high rate to allow trials to be of smaller size and shorter duration than are required for studies of cancer.

Adenomatous polyps in the colon or rectum may be suitable endpoints as there is suggestive, though not conclusive, evidence that such polyps may be precursors for malignant disease (Day and Morson 1978; Correa 1978). In individuals who have had an adenomatous polyp removed by polypectomy, additional polyps are seen on colonoscopy after two years in over 20 percent of patients (Henry et al 1975). This rate of recurrence is sufficiently high that dietary intervention trials can be conducted using several hundred patients with adenomatous polyps over a period of two years. Since patients with familial polyposis are at high risk of cancer, regression of rectal polyps in such patients has also been used as an endpoint for a trial of vitamin supplementation (Bussey et al 1982).

The relevance of studies based on polyps to the prevention of colon cancer depends, of course, on the assumption that they are precursors for malignant disease. While this is widely accepted, the association will not be conclusively proven until randomized trials have established that the removal of polyps prevents malignant disease. At present, it remains possible that polyps and cancer have one or more etiologic factors in common but that cancer does not necessarily develop from polyps, just as chronic bronchitis and lung cancer share smoking as an etiologic factor, but chronic bronchitis is not a precursor for malignant disease. In this situation, trials which were able to demonstrate that the rate of polyp occurrence could be reduced by dietary means would have direct relevance to cancer in establishing that the dietary manipulation was feasible - an important step when major alterations in diet such as reduction of fat consumption or increase in fibre consumption are required - but inferences about the relationship between diet and cancer would be indirect and rest on the assumption that polyps and cancer have a common cause. In contrast, if a trial which employed the recurrence of a precursor lesion as the clinical endpoint failed to detect an effect of a dietary intervention, it could be argued that the intervention had been attempted too late in development of the disease process to be effective, particularly if the dietary intervention were expected to effect initiation rather than promotion. Randomized trials which employ cancer as an endpoint will ultimately be required to establish that dietary interventions can prevent malignant disease.

Cellular events may be the earliest markers of a disease process and may therefore be suitable as short-term assays to test dietary intervention strategies, though the link with malignant disease would clearly need to be established. Damaged nuclei are seen in animals after exposure to several colon carcinogens (Wargovich et al 1983b), as well as to some toxic agents (Duncan and Heddle 1984), and are also seen in human colon biopsies (Ronen et al 1983). Epithelial damage followed by increased cell proliferation has been seen in animals after exposure to bile acids and fatty acids (Wargovich et al 1983a; Bird et al 1984), and it has been suggested that this damage might be related to the promoting effect of fat in the colon (Newmark et al 1984). These lesions, or other cellular endpoints, such as measures of cell kinetics, could be used as endpoints of dietary trials in circumstances in which the conducting of a biopsy of the colon was both ethical and feasible, such as during colonoscopy.

PRESENT AND FUTURE TRIALS

A number of randomized trials are either in progress or are being planned which employ cancer, polyps or cellular events as clinical endpoints to test the major dietary factors which have been hypothesized to be protective against colon cancer. These include dietary supplementation with beta-carotene, vitamins C and E, increased dietary fibre, and decreased dietary fat. Incidence of cancers of all sites, including the colon, is being examined as part of a study of American physicians in a trial of supplementation with beta-carotene (Richard Peto, personal communication). The rates of occurrence of adenomatous polyps in persons who have had previous adenomas removed during colonoscopy are being examined in several studies in Australia, the United States and Canada. After initial polypectomy, patients are random-ized into one or more dietary intervention arms and are reexamined at intervals up to three years to ascertain the occurrence of new polyps. Supplementation with beta-carotene is being compared with a placebo in such trials in Australia (Robert MacLennon, personal communication) and the U.S.A. (Phyllis Bowen, personal communication), and supplementation with a combination of vitamins C and E is under investigation in Canada (Bruce et al 1981). The separate and combined effects of all three vitamins are also being evaluated in an investigation in the U.S.A. in which subjects are allocated to one of four groups, with or without supplements of beta-carotene and with or without supplements of vitamins C and E in combination (John Barron, personal communication). Alteration of dietary macronutrients is also under investigation. We are comparing the occurrence rate of polyps in patients who receive monthly counseling on a high fibre-low fat diet containing at least 50 g of total energy taken as fat, with that in patients who are counseled every four months on a control diet following Canada's Food Guide which includes an average of less than 20 g of fibre and 75-120 g of fat. Regression of rectal polyps in patients with familial polyposis has been studied in relation to vitamin C supplementation (Bussey et al 1982) and a comparable study of increased fibre consumption, together with vitamin C and E supplementation, is now underway (Jerome De Cosse, personal communication). Cell kinetics have also been studied in patients with familial polyposis in relation to vitamin C supplementation (Bussey et al 1982), and rates of nuclear and epithelial damage are being compared in biopsy specimens obtained from healthy volunteers who consume either a high-fat diet containing about 250 g of fat or a low-fat diet containing 25 g of fat (H. Himal, personal communication).

The testing of current or new dietary hypotheses in a series of intervention trials should make it possible to establish whether dietary changes are feasible and should clarify the role of dietary factors in the prevention of cancer of the colon. Trials employing a precursor lesion as the endpoint can establish that long term dietary interventions have no significant side effects and that compliance is appropriately high, as well as explore the possibility that diet can influence the development of disease. Finally, large long term trials using cancer incidence or mortality as the clinical endpoint can test the ability of dietary interventions to prevent malignant disease.

CURRENT DIETARY RECOMMENDATIONS

Until the results of future research are available, recommendations on diet must be based on a synthesis of current knowledge of the relationship between diet and cancer. The National Academy of Sciences recently published interim dietary guidelines (Grobstein et al 1982) recommending that the consumption of fat be reduced in the average American diet, stressing the importance of fruits, vegetables and whole grain cereal products, recommending minimal consumption of foods preserved by salt curing or smoking, encouraging efforts to identify mutagens in foods, proposing that efforts continue to minimize contamination of foods with carcinogens and recommending that alcoholic beverages be consumed only in moderation. It was stressed that "the weight of evidence suggests that what we eat during our lifetime strongly influences the probability of developing certain kinds of cancer, but that it is not now possible, and may never be possible, to specify a diet that protects all people against all forms of cancer." Such dietary recommendations will need to be reviewed as new evidence becomes available but, despite their necessarily tentative nature, they form the basis of a nutritionally sound diet which has, on present evidence, the potential for reducing cancer rates in North America.

REFERENCES

Armstrong B, Doll R (1975). Environmental factors and cancer incidence and mortality in different countries, with special reference to dietary practices. Br J Cancer 15:617.

Bird RP, Medline A, Furrer R, Bruce WR (1984). Orally administered fat can produce readily visualized damage to the colonic epithelium of mice. Unpublished observation.

Bruce WR, McKeown-Eyssen G, Ciampi A, Dion PW, Boyd N (1981). Strategies for dietary intervention studies in colon cancer. Cancer 47:1121.

Bussey HJR, DeCosse JJ, Deschner EE, Eyser AA, Lesser ML, Borson BC, Ritchie SM, Thompson JPS, Wadsworth J (1982). A randomized trial of ascorbic acid in polyposis coli. Cancer 50:1434.

Correa P (1978). Epidemiology of polyps and cancer. In Morson BC (ed): "The Pathogenesis of Colorectal Cancer", Philadelphia: W.B. Saunders, p. 126.

Dales LG, Friedman GD, Ury HK, Grossman S, Williams SR (1978). A case-control study of relationships of diet and other traits to colorectal cancer in American Blacks. Am J Epidemiol 109:132.

Day DW, Morson BD (1978). The adenoma-carcinoma sequence. In Morson BC (ed): "The Pathogenesis of Colorectal Cancer", Philadelphia: WB Saunders, p. 58.

Duncan AMV, Heddle JA (1984). The frequency and distribution of apoptosis induced by non-carcinogenic agents in mouse colonic crypts. Cancer Letters, in press.

Graham S, Dayal H, Swanson M, Mittelman A, Wilkinson G (1978). Diet in the epidemiology of cancer of the colon and rectum. J Natl Cancer Inst 61:709.

Grobstein C, Cairns J. Berliner R. Broitman SA, Campbell TC, Gussow JD, Kolonel LN, Kirtchevsky D, Mertz W, Miller AB, Prival MJ, Slaga T, Wattenberg L, Sugimura T (1982). "Diet, Nutrition, and Cancer." Washington: National Academy Press.

Henry LG, Condon RE, Schulte WJ, Aprahamian C, DeCosse JJ (1975). Risk of recurrence of colon polyps. Ann Surg 182:511.

Higginson J (1966). Etiological factors in gastrointestinal cancer in man. J Natl Cancer Inst 37:527.

Jain M, Cook GM, David FG, Grace MG, Howe GR, Miller AB (1980). A case-control study of diet and colorectal cancer. Int J Cancer 26:757.

Knox EG (1977). Foods and diseases. Br J Prev Soc Med 31:71.

McKeown-Eyssen GE, Bruce WR (1984). Approaches to an understanding of the relation between diet and colon cancer. Unpublished data.

McKeown-Eyssen GE, Thomas DC. Sample size determination in case-control studies: The influence of the distribution of exposure. Unpublished data.

Modan B, Barell V, Lubin F, Modan M, Greenberg RA, Graham S (1975). Low-fiber intake as an etiologic factor in cancer of the colon. J Natl Cancer Inst 55:15.

Newmark HL, Wargovich MJ, Bruce WR (1984). Colon cancer and dietary fat, phosphate and calcium: A hypothesis. J Natl Cancer Inst 72:1323.

Phillips RL (1975). Role of life-style and dietary habits in risk of cancer among Seventh-Day Adventists. Cancer Res 35:3513.

Ronen A, Heddle JA, DUncan AMV (1983). Site specificity in the induction of nuclear anomalies by carcinogens. Ann NY Acad Sci 407:479.

Wargovich MJ, Eng VWS, Newmark HL, Bruce WR (1983a). Calcium ameliorates the toxic effect of deoxycholic acid on colonic epithelium. Carcinogenesis 4:1205.

Wargovich MJ, Goldberg MT, Newmark HL, Bruce WR (1983b). Nuclear aberrations as a short-term test for genotoxicity to the colon: evaluation of nineteen agents in mice. J Natl Cancer Inst 71:133.

Carcinoma of the Large Bowel and Its Precursors, pages 285–296
© 1985 Alan R. Liss, Inc.

STRATEGIES AND RATIONALE FOR INTERVENTION STUDIES

Bandaru S. Reddy, DVM, Ph.D.
Division of Nutrition ad Endocrinology
Naylor Dana Institute for Disease Prevention
American Health Foundation
Valhalla, New York 10595

Cancer of the colon is one of the most prevalent cancers in the western world, accounting for more than 130,000 new cases with about 50% mortality rate each year in the United States, and exhibiting more than a tenfold excess when compared to the rural populations in Africa, Asia, and South America (American Cancer Society 1984; Correa and Haenszel 1978; Burkitt 1978; Jensen 1983). In addition, there are subgroups in the population at increased risk for large bowel cancer which include patients with prior adenomas, ulcerative colitis of more than seven years duration, a family history of one of the polyposis syndromes, or inherited non-polyposis colon cancer syndromes (Winawer 1984).

Prevention of colon cancer could be achieved through primary and secondary prevention. Primary prevention includes the identification of risk factors responsible for colon cancer and their eradication, whereas the secondary prevention includes the early detection of colon cancer prior to its more advanced form as well as detection and eradication of premalignant conditions before they are transformed or progress into cancer (Winawer 1984). The desirable goals of any colon cancer prevention program are to emphasize both primary and secondary prevention.

During the last fifteen years, a substantial amount of progress has been made in understanding the relationship between dietary components and the development of colon cancer in man. The data base is sufficiently convincing with respect to a promoting effect of total dietary fat and a protective effect of certain dietary fibers and micronutrients in colon cancer (National Research Council 1982; Doll and Peto 1981; Wynder 1975; Reddy 1982; Jensen et al 1982). Current research also suggests that these nutritional factors may operate largely during the post-initiating stage of carcinogenesis and have a preponderant influence on the eventual outcome of the neoplastic process in man. It is believed that the same factors that affect colon cancer incidence in the general population also influence the recurrence of adenomatous polyps after polypectomy and their trans-formation into carcinomas of the colon, recurrence of colon carcinomas after surgical intervention in cancer patients, and the symptomatic and asymptomatic individuals affected with the autosomal dominantly inherited non-polyposis colorectal cancer syndrome. Dietary inter-vention in these patients should result in objective increase in disease-free survival and an overall reduction in the mortality from this disease or its recurrence.

RATIONALE FOR COLON CANCER PREVENTION BY DIETARY MODIFI-CATION

The research in the area of nutrition and cancer has developed into a body of information that now enables rational approaches to primary and secondary prevention. The first report of the National Academy of Sciences Committee on Diet, Nutrition, and Cancer identified sev-eral dietary risk factors as well as protective factors for colon cancer (National Research Council 1982). This suggestion came from epidemiologic studies of dietary intake in human populations either with or at risk for the development of colon cancer and from laboratory animal studies. The following discussion will evaluate some of the evidence suggesting that nutritional factors have a role in primary and secondary prevention of colon cancer in humans.

Evidence from Epidemiologic Studies:

Available evidence reviewed by Doll and Peto (1981) indicates that through dietary modification we might achieve a 90% reduction of large bowel cancer mortality. These data were derived from epidemiologic studies which yielded estimations of relative risk and population attributable risk, and from viewing the extremes of colon cancer incidence and mortality rates throughout the world.

It is not the purpose of this paper to recite the evidence from human nutritional epidemiologic studies, but to evaluate the scientific evidence for a dietary etiology of colon cancer. Several descriptive epidemiologic studies have found a positive association between colon cancer mortality or incidence in different countries and per capita availability of total fat (Armstrong and Doll 1975; Carroll and Khor 1975), and animal fat (Drasar and Irving 1973; Howel 1975) estimated from food balance sheets. The statistical correlation of the incidence of colon cancer and prevalence of non-hereditary adenomatous polyps has been documented (Correa et al 1972). The incidence of adenomatous polyps is prevalant in the upper social class in Cali, Colombia, who consume westernized food (Correa 1975). Such interventional correlations should be interpreted with caution because the dietary data were based not on actual intake information, but on food disappearance data (McKeown-Eyssen 1983). These correlation studies were based on populations rather than on individuals. In addition, there were differences from country to country in accuracy with the data that were calculated.

The nutritional epidemiologic studies turned to case-control comparisons and prospective studies in order to define more accurately the etiologic factors. These studies demonstrated an association between colon cancer risk and dietary beef (Haenszel et al 1973; Mannous et al 1983), total fat (Jain et al 1970; West et al 1983; Wynder 1975), and saturated fat (Wynder 1975; Miller et al 1983). In another study, no association was observed within countries between regional or ethnic colon cancer rates and meat and fat (Kolonel et al 1981). These conflicting results could be explained on the basis that several of these studies neglected to take into consideration the other confounding factors, such as the intake of dietary fiber, cruciferous vegetables, and other food items that have been shown to reduce the risk of colon cancer (Jensen et al 1982; Reddy et al 1978; Graham et al 1978). Several of these studies have combined cases of colon and rectal cancer, despite the evidence that these conditions do not share the identical etiology. In a study of cases and hospital controls among Blacks in California, Dales et al (1979) observed a direct association between risk of colon cancer and frequent consumption of foods high in saturated fat. The association was strongest for those who consumed diets high in saturated fat and low in fiber content.

Recently, attention has been directed toward the protective effect of dietary fiber, which generally includes indigestable carbohydrates and carbohydrate-like components of food, such as cellulose, lignin, hemicelluloses, pentosans, gums, and pectin. The major categories of foods that provide dietary fiber are whole-grain cereals, vegetables, and fruits.

Attempts to correlate the fiber content of diets with colon cancer risk have yielded mixed results because certain of these findings may have arisen, at least in part, from methodological limitations of these studies. Inconclusive results of early correlation studies in relation to dietary fiber could be explained by the fact that the statistics of dietary fiber were based on estimates of crude fiber intake or crude fiber disappearance data (Drasar and Irving 1973), and these calculations underestimate the intake of total dietary fiber. Consequently, early reports provided incomplete data on the amount and type of fiber consumed.

Recent studies comparing rural and urban populations in Denmark, Finland, and Sweden and urban population in New York indicated that the rural Scandinavians consumed more total dietary fiber and whole-grain cereals than the urban populations (Jensen et al 1982; Domellof et al 1982; Reddy 1982), although all populations were on high-fat diets. A case-control study also found that the consumption of high-fiber foods by colon cancer cases was significantly lower than that of controls, but there was no difference between rectal cancer cases and controls (Modan et al 1975). Attempts to correlate the fiber content of diets with genotoxic compounds (carcinogens and mutagens) in the colonic contents and colon cancer risk of populations in Kuopio and Helsinki, Finland have provided interesting results. Our recent data indicate that the healthy individuals from Kuopio and Helsinki exhibiting high fecal mutagenic activity are somewhat different from those showing little or no mutagenic activity with respect to intake of food items such as whole-grain cereals and breads. The individuals excreting high levels of mutagens in the feces were consuming diets low in these high-fibrous food items (Table 1). These findings lend support to the hypothesis that dietary fiber plays a protective role in colon carcinogenesis.

Table 1

Dietary Fat and Fiber Intake and Fecal Mutagenic Activity in Finnish Populations

Grams/day			Mutation ratio[a]			
Fiber		Total Fat	TA 100		TA 98	
Whole grain and cereal	Total fiber		+S9	−S9	+S9	−S9
22.5	38.6	108	< 3	< 3	< 3	< 3
12.3	20.5	118	11.4	7.4	9.7	12.1

[a] Fecal sample with mutation ratio less than 3 is considered inactive.

Very few epidemiologic studies have been conducted to determine the relationship between micronutrients and the incidence of colon cancer in humans. This is due partly to the difficulty of identifying populations with significantly different intakes of these nutrients. The epidemiologic evidence relating colon cancer to dietary selenium is limited by suggestion (Griffin 1979). Epidemiologic studies suggest that the amount of selenium in soil and forage crops varied inversely with colon cancer incidence in a wide variety of countries. However, in certain geographic areas, such as Finland, where the soil is deficient in selenium, the low incidence of colon cancer may be explained in part on the fact that the Finns consume diets high in cereal fiber (Reddy et al 1978; Jensen et al 1982). Thus, in Finland, the selenium effects on colon cancer are likely to be influenced by other factors, e.g., dietary fiber. Studies using laboratory animal models suggest that selenium-mediated inhibition of colon carcinogenesis appears to be effective during and before carcinogen treatment (initiation phase), but not during the post-initiation phase of carcinogenesis (Jacobs et al 1981). A major concern with selenium is its narrow range of toxicity. Toxic reproductive and teratogenic effects of selenium have been reported for both animals and man (Buell 1983). Additional investigative effort is required to effectively study the potential of selenium as a modifier of carcinogenesis.

Vitamin E is an important intracellular antioxidant and theoretically could inhibit colon carcinogenesis through decreased lipid peroxidation and/or increased detoxification of carcinogenic substances. There is also a possibility that vitamin E may have an effect on the metabolism of selenium. However, there have been no reported epidemiologic studies correlating vitamin E consumption and international colon cancer incidence rates. Because vitamin E is present in a variety of commonly eaten foods, it is difficult to identify population groups with substantially different levels of intake. However, frequent consumption of cruciferous vegetables has been associated inversely in case-control and cohort studies with cancer of the colon (Graham et al 1978). A number of compounds inhibiting chemically-induced carcinogenesis in laboratory animals are present in cruciferous vegetables and include aromatic isothiocyanates, indoles, and phenols (Wattenberg 1983). Investigators have not yet established which of these compounds may be responsible for the protective effects observed in epidemiological studies.

STRATEGIES AND PROSPECTS FOR PRIMARY AND SECONDARY PREVENTION OF COLON CANCER

What can be done to reduce mortality from colon cancer by taking advantage of current knowledge? What other kinds of information need to be generated to promote control of colon cancer?

During the last decade, a substantial amount of progress has been made in understanding the relationship between dietary constituents and the development of colon cancer in man. The data base is sufficiently convincing with respect to enhancment of colon cancer as a function of total fat intake and protection by certain dietary fibers. The populations with high incidence of colon cancer are characterized by consumption of high dietary fat which may be a risk factor in the absence of factors that are protective, such as the use of whole-grain cereals, high fibrous foods and vegetables - mainly the cruciferous vegetables. Application of the findings made thus far in colon cancer research to the general public should, therefore, have a far-reaching impact on the major diseases of the western world.

Current research in animal models, which suggests that the carcinogenic response to a variety of colon carcinogens is enhanced by dietary fat and inhibited by several dietary fibers, indicates that these nutritional factors may operate during the promotional phase of carcinogenesis. The carcinogenic process in humans may have similar characteristics. The fact that ubiquitous environmental carcinogens are present at very low concentrations and the extent of the carcinogenic stress from this source is probably rather weak, suggests that promoting factors may have a preponderant influence on the eventual outcome of the neoplastic process in humans. The understanding of post-initiation events appears to offer some promise that intervention in the cancer process in man prior to the occurrence of overt tumors may be an achievable and realistic goal. Because promotion of post-initiation events is a reversible process, in contrast to the rapid irreversible or long-lasting process of initiation by carcinogens, manipulation of promotion would appear to be the ideal method of colon cancer prevention. However, in prevention, it makes little difference by what mechanism an agent operates, provided that its partial or total elimination can be shown to lead to a decline in cancer incidence. In this regard, advice to the public at large assumes particular importance because several decades may span the gap between initiation and the clinical manifestation of cancer. Therefore, steps taken today may have a major impact on the outcome of future events.

If the hypothesis is correct that the same factors affecting colon cancer incidence also influence the recurrence of adenomatous polyps after polypectomy, transformation of adenomas into carcinomas of the colon, and recurrence of colon carcinomas after surgical intervention in cancer patients, then dietary intervention in these patients should result in objective increase in disease-free survival and improved overall survival. The same benefits should hold also for the symptomatic and asymptomatic patients affected with autosomal dominantly inherited non-polyposis colorectal cancer syndromes which may account for as much as 5-7% of all occurrences of colorectal cancer. The overall goal is to reduce the incidence of colon cancer in these high-risk groups. We suggest that randomized prospective clinical trials be conducted in patients at high risk for carcinomas of the colon with the aim of reducing the incidence of new polyps or carcinomas. These clinical trials will not only address issues of specificity not resolved in epidemiologic studies and the clinical relevance of animal models, but will also evaluate participant acceptance of the intervention.

These prudent measures for the general population as well as patients or families at high risk for colon cancer development are imperative when various lines of evidence are concordant and point to current dietary patterns in the United States and western countries which have an elevated risk for colon cancer. The advantage of encouraging the public to alter their dietary pattern is that these measures have no obvious adverse effects. Therefore, these dietary recommendations - namely, lower total fat intake and increased consumption of dietary fiber - can be made without concern for incurring any adverse effects as might be found with a drug-oriented management and disease prevention program. Hence, in terms of prevention of colon cancer, a decision to alter dietary habits leading to a lower intake of dietary fat and higher intake of certain dietary fibers has potential beneficial effects which go beyond colon cancer in that a reduction in fat intake might also influence the risk for other diet-related cancer and, in particular, could reduce the rate of coronary heart disease.

Planning and evaluation of clinical trials in patients with early stages of primary cancer must clearly recognize that the intervention will usually not test an effect on the early or initiation phase of carcinogenesis since this early stage has already been passed and cancer has already developed. Rather, this population of patients would be a model for testing inhibition or reversal of the later phase (promotion) of carcinogenesis. The patients with non-hereditary adenomatous polyps and members of hereditary colon cancer-prone families also fall into this category.

The significance of the proposed dietary modifications lies in its ability to provide information relevant to the use of dietary intervention as a form of totally effective nontoxic therapy for patients with colon cancer and adenomatous polyps. These recommendations apply to the public at large.

The modified dietary regimen consists of a reduction of dietary fat to 25% of fat calories with a polyunsaturated, saturated, and monounsaturated fatty acid ratio of 1:1:1 and an increase in complex carbohydrate intake. Total dietary fiber intake per day should be increased to 36g based on McCance and Widdowson's fiber values (Paul and Southgate 1978) which is approximately 25g of neutral detergent fiber. It has been shown that a moderate reduction of the dietary fat intake of 20% to 25% of total calories does not appear to constitute a health risk if an adequate ratio of polyunsaturated:saturated fatty acids is maintained (Judd et al 1983). There is concern about the fat-soluble vitamin intake since the level of intake would result in the intake of fat-soluble vitamins, mainly vitamin A. The fatty foods are replaced by those rich in complex carbohydrates from products of vegetable origin which are a good source of vitamin A precursors, the carotenes. There is also a concern that high-fiber diets have some effect on the availability of certain nutrients in the body, particularly minerals. Diets containing less than 25g of neutral detergent fiber and fat at 20% or more of the total calories can be considered safe (Judd et al 1983).

In order to achieve the above objective, we recommend eating fewer foods high in saturated and unsaturated fats and to increase the consumption of fruits, vegetables, and whole-grain cereal products daily. These vegetables should include dark green leafy vegetables, carrots, winter squash, tomatoes, cabbage, cauliflower, and Brussel sprouts, to cite a few. This is not a diet which we generally adopt as an emergency measure after we have indulged in nutritional excesses, but rather represents a continuing life-long, low-risk, yet pleasant, tasteful, and nutritious diet from the public health point of view. Therefore, the time to make nutritional declarations to western populations is now. The oncologists will have the opportunity to monitor the success of such nutritional modification.

ACKNOWLEDGEMENTS

This research was supported in part from grants CA-29602, CA-17613 and CA-32617, and contracts CP-85659 from the National Cancer Institute. The author acknowledges the expert assistance of Ms. Arlene Banow in preparation of the manuscript.

REFERENCES

American Cancer Society, Inc. Cancer Facts and Figures. New York, 1984.

Armstrong D, Doll R (1975). Environmental factors and cancer incidence and mortality in different countries, with special reference to dietary practices. Int J Cancer 15:617.

Buell DN (1983). Potential hazards of selenium as a chemopreventive agent. Seminars in Oncology 10:311.

Burkitt DP (1978). Colorectal cancer: Fiber and other dietary factors. Am J Clin Nutr 31:S58.

Carroll KK, Khor HT (1975). Dietary fat in relation to tumorigenesis. Prog Biochem Pharmacol 10:308.

Correa P (1975). Comments on the epidemiology of large bowel cancer. Cancer Res 35:3395.

Correa P, Duque E, Cuello C, Haenszel W (1972). Polyps of the colon and rectum in Cali, Columbia. Int J Cancer 9:86.

Correa P, Haenszel W (1978). The epidemiology of large bowel cancer. Adv Cancer Res 26:1.

Dales IG, Friedman GD, Wry HK et al (1979). Case control study of relationship of diet and other traits to colorectal cancer in American Blacks. Am J Epidemiol 109:132.

Doll R, Peto R (1981). The causes of cancer: Quantitative estimates of avoidable risks of cancer in the United States today. J Natl Cancer Inst 66:1192.

Domellof L, Darby L, Hanson D, Simi B, Reddy BS (1982). Fecal sterols and bacterial B-glucuronidase activity: A preliminary study of healthy volunteers from Umea, Sweden, and metropolitan New York. Nutr Cancer 4:120.

Drasar BS, Irving D (1973). Experimental factors and cancer of the colon and breast. Br J Cancer 27:167.

Graham S, Dayal H, Swanson M (1978). Diet in the epidemiology of cancer of the colon and rectum. J Natl Cancer Inst 61:709.

Griffin AB (1979). Role of selenium in the chemoprevent-
ion of cancer. Adv Cancer Res 29:419.
Howell MA (1975). Diet as an etiological factor in the
development of cancers of colon and rectum. J Chron
Diseases 28:67.
Jacobs MM, Frost CF, Beam FA (1981). Biochemical and
clinical effects of selenium on dimethylhydrazine-
induced colon cancer in rats. Cancer Res 41:4458.
Jensen OM (1983). Colon cancer epidemiology. In Autrup
H. Williams GM (eds): "Experimental Colon Carcino-
genesis", CRC Press, Boca Raton, FL, pp 3.
Jensen OM, MacLennan R, Wahrendorf J (1982). Diet, bowel
function, fecal characteristics and large bowel cancer
in Denmark and Finland. Nutr Cancer 4:5.
Judd JT, Kelsay JL, Mertz W (1983). Potential risks from
low-fat diets. Seminars in Oncology 10:273.
Kolonel LN, Hankin JH, Lee J, Chu SY, Nomura AMY, Ward
Hinds M (1981). Nutrient intakes in relation to cancer
incidence in Hawaii. Br J Cancer 44:132.
McKeown-Eyssen G (1983). A diet to prevent colon cancer:
How do we get there from here. In Roe DA (ed): "Diet,
Nutrition, and Cancer: From Basic Research to Policy
Implications", Alan R. Liss Inc., New York, pp 243.
Miller AB, Howe GR, Jain M (1983). Food items and food
groups as risk factors in a case-control study of diet
and colorectal cancer. Int J Cancer 32:155.
Modan B, Barell V, Lubin F, Modan M, Greenburg RA, Graham
S (1975). Low-fiber intake as an etiologic factor in
cancer of the colon. J Natl Cancer Inst 55:15.
National Research Council (1982). "Diet, Nutrition, and
Cancer", National Academy Press, Washington, DC.
Paul AA, Southgate DAT (1978). "McCance and Widdowson's,
The Composition of Foods," HMSO, London.
Reddy BS (1982). Dietary fiber and colon carciogenesis.
A Critical review. In Vahouny G, Kritchevsky D (eds):
"Dietary Fiber in Health and Disease", Plenum Press, New
York, p 265.
Reddy BS, Hedges AR, Laakso K, Synder EL (1978).
Metabolic epidemiology of large bowel cancer. Fecal
bulk and constituents of high-risk North American and
low-risk Finnish population. Cancer 42:2382.
Wattenberg LW (1983). Inhibition of neoplasia by minor
dietary constituents. Cancer Res 43:2448S.

Winawer SJ (1984). Introduction to position papers from
  the Third International Symposium on Colorectal Cancer.
  Ca-A Cancer Journal for Clinicnas 34:130.
Wynder EL (1975). The epidemiology of large bowel cancer.
  Cancer Res 35:3388.

Index